The Brain Health Workbook

The Brain Health Workbook

Build a brain that supports everything you want to do and be!

Jean Courtney

This book is for informational purposes only. It is not intended to serve as a substitute for professional medical advice. The author and publisher specifically disclaim any and all liability arising directly or indirectly from the use of any information contained in this book. A health care professional should be consulted regarding your specific medical situation.

The Brain Health Workbook

1st Edition 2026

ADVANCE PRAISE

"Wellness has been a focus of mine for nearly a century. Jean Courtney's book gives a great daily blueprint for its main components."

— ***Deborah Szekely,*** *Founder Rancho La Puerta and The Golden Door, Premier Destination Spa Resorts*

"I love Jean Courtney's practical approach to clearing your body and mind for a healthier brain. Not only does she deliver you practical recipes for eliminating toxic foods but daily meditations to ditch the thoughts that go along with them. The recipes are delicious, doable, and inspire you to make long-term changes in the way you think and eat."

— ***Emily Morse,*** *Doctor of Human Sexuality, Founder, Sex With Emily*

"When healthy eating is this delicious, there's no reason not to! The simple, easy- to-follow recipes in this cookbook are delicious. And the nutritional power packed into each recipe is doctor-approved. This is an easy prescription to make!"

— ***Dr. Erica Oberg, ND MPH,*** *Integrative Natural Medicine, Functional Medicine & Regenerative Anti-Aging Therapies*

"A great primer on how diet affects the brain, a topic we simply don't discuss enough, with inventive, yet easy to follow recipes."

— ***Kathleen Flinn,*** *author of 2007* New York Times *bestseller,* The Sharper Your Knife, the Less You Cry.

For my beautiful Mom, Zita.

Dementia changed her life as she knew it and taught me more than I ever thought I would need to know.

Her memories left her, functions followed one by one, and finally her body gave out fully. But her happy spirit remains ALWAYS.

— Jean Courtney

AUTHOR'S NOTE

Hello! You might be wondering WHY a non-medical professional wrote this book.

Welllllll... it was because so many people asked for it.

One cooking class participant in her 80's said to me... HURRY UP AND GET A BOOK OUT! I need it and am running out of time!

So here it is.

I am a retired legal investigator whose mom got dementia. I worked at a fast-paced, busy law firm and watched many of the people around me succumb to stress. Marriages ended, tempers were short, people got sick.

I decided I didn't want to spend my "one wild and precious life" living that way. I made the conscious decision to choose time and health over the good salary I had.

Sooooo.....I figured I should use my research skills to study health with all the time I had gifted myself, since I wasn't going to have a lot of money to pay for health issues.

I started studying ways to optimize and maximize my own health - that led me down the path of the microbiome, epigenetics, all sorts of things.

And then my mom got dementia in her 70's. It devastated my family on many levels. I tried, but it was too late to help her.

I wanted to do all I could to help myself and others with dementia in their families.

I started teaching cooking classes at Rancho La Puerta, a wellness resort, on foods for brain health, then from that started giving talks and workshops about lifestyle factors for brain health, and this book was the logical next step.

INTRODUCTION

YOUR BRAIN

It is the center for all your past memories, present thoughts, and future decisions.

This 3 pound ball of wonder contains billions of neurons and hundreds of miles of blood vessels. It is one of busiest and most complex parts of your body.

Do you want to maximize your best asset?

When you shift your mindset to think of your brain as THE MOST IMPORTANT part of you, the thing that makes unique YOU operate in YOUR unique way, it will be easy to make decisions that benefit your brain.

Think of your brain as a bank — the more you invest now, the more you will have to withdraw from later.

And good news: what benefits your brain later also benefits your body now!

If you have a brain, you have a risk for dementia.

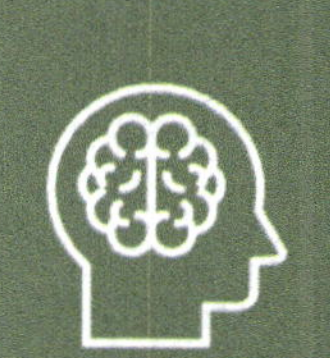

Your Brain is You!

You want it to be vibrant, alive, and full of joy!

INTRODUCTION

Dementia is a syndrome leading to deterioration of cognitive function.

This cognitive decline affects memory and daily activities such as driving, cooking, and hygiene.

There are several types of dementia, including Alzheimer's, vascular, lewy body, and frontotemporal.

Worldwide, approximately 55 million people suffer from dementia.

This is projected to increase to 78 million by 2030, and more than double to 139 million by 2050.

Rates are 60% higher in women than men.

This devastating syndrome takes a huge toll on patients and their families — emotional, physical, and financial.

Care costs average $8,000-$9,000 per month for memory care facilities. This number goes up to $12,000+ if the person becomes nonambulatory

The global cost was estimated at $1.3 trillion in 2019, and forecasted to rise to $2.8 trillion by 2030.

We have a shortage of dementia care specialists, so this will add to the burden of already overtaxed primary care physicians.

Pharmacology currently has no cure for dementia.

What we have right now are proven lifestyle factors that help minimize the risk of cognitive decline. Those are what we will focus on here.

LIFESTYLE FACTORS

Let's focus on lifestyle factors to support your brain health:

FOOD — the software that runs your body's hardware

THOUGHTS — create hormones that impact your body processes

EXERCISE — activates blood flow to your brain

SLEEP — a nightly dishwasher for your brain

CONNECTION — critical to combat isolation and loneliness

CURIOSITY — stimulates brain engagement and learning

FOOD

We think of food as fuel.

Let's shift our mindset to think of food as **information** for our bodies. Every single process that happens in your body is driven by nutrients.

Nutrients are vitamins and minerals that act as building blocks for your brain and body.

Food is constantly EDUCATING our cells (positively and negatively) to drive each and every one of our body's processes.

Good information provides good outcome.

Food is the software that runs your body's hardware.

At 3 lbs, your brain is about 2% of your body's overall weight, but it uses about 20% of the energy generated by the foods you choose to eat.

When it comes to providing your brain with good information to feed your cells, what you take OUT is as important as what you put IN.

FOOD

What to take **OUT**	What to put **IN**
☐ Sugar	☐ Organic clean whole food
☐ White Flour	☐ Large variety of fruits and vegetables... your brain loves flavonoids and phytonutrients
☐ Ultra-processed Foods	☐ Cruciferous vegetables and leafy greens
☐ CONVENTIONAL meat, dairy, and seafood (this means NOT organic, grass-fed, pasture raised, wild caught)	☐ Coconut and almond flours
☐ Most vegetable oils	☐ Clean organic, fresh olive oil, avocado oil, coconut oil
	☐ Beneficial spices — turmeric, cinnamon, ginger, oregano, cumin
	☐ Clean fatty fish, i.e. Salmon
	☐ Raw organic nuts
	☐ Avocados
	☐ Berries, especially blueberries and strawberries
	☐ Cacao

FOOD

We generally eat at least three times every day. There are a LOT of chances to get it *right*.

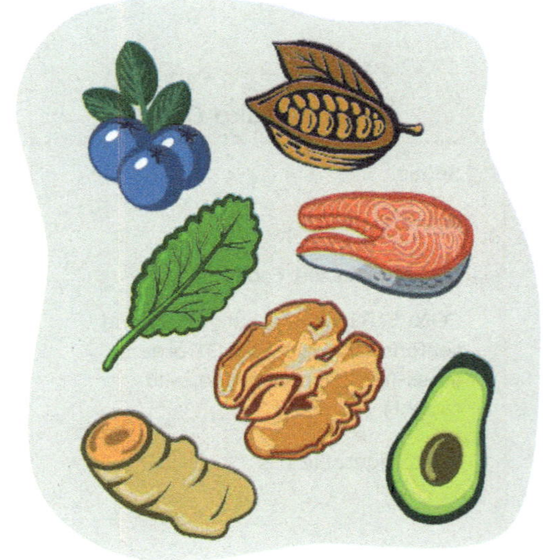

CONSTRUCT A DIET RICH IN:

Phytochemicals: chemical compounds produced by plants to help them resist bacteria/infection

Flavonoids: help regulate cellular activity and fight off free radicals that cause oxidative stress/imbalance

Antioxidants: help fight free radicals

THE MICROBIOME

Your gut microbiome is the ecosystem of bacteria that live in your intestines.

There are approximately 100 trillion microbes in the human gut.

The best way to keep these bacteria happy is to feed them a variety of foods. Your microbiome loves diversity.

You can increase the diversity when you build your yogurt for breakfast, your salad for lunch, and your bowl for dinner.

Add in as many different ingredients as you want. Remember, food is **INFORMATION** for your body and all of its processes. Every process uses different information. That's why variety is key.

THE MICROBIOME

Tips to make it easier to keep your yogurt, salads, dinner bowls full of easily accessible variety:

- Once a week, grind chia and flax seeds. Mix them in a jar with hemp seeds and keep in your refrigerator door.
- Blend collagen and cacao powders and keep in a jar in the pantry.
- Put the spices you use frequently (cinnamon, turmeric, black pepper) in an easily accessible spot (not on a spice rack where you have to search them out).
- Freeze a small piece of ginger

You don't need large quantities of any one thing. ***Smaller doses of a variety of nutrients feed different bacteria.*** Make it as easy as possible to add variety to your meals.

BUILD YOUR YOGURT

ORGANIC FULL FAT GREEK YOGURT

- ☐ CHIA SEEDS
- ☐ FLAX SEEDS
- ☐ HEMP SEEDS
- ☐ BANANA (FROZEN WORKS)
- ☐ BLUEBERRIES
- ☐ STRAWBERRIES
- ☐ RASPBERRIES
- ☐ BLACKBERRIES
- ☐ PEACHES
- ☐ PERSIMMONS
- ☐ ALMONDS
- ☐ PECANS
- ☐ WALNUTS
- ☐ SUNFLOWER SEEDS
- ☐ PEPITAS
- ☐ HONEY
- ☐ CINNAMON
- ☐ COLLAGEN POWDER
- ☐ CACAO POWDER
- ☐ CACAO NIBS

BUILD YOUR SALAD

- ☐ KALE
- ☐ WATERCRESS
- ☐ ARUGULA
- ☐ ROMAINE
- ☐ BUTTER LETTUCE
- ☐ DANDELION GREENS
- ☐ CABBAGE (RED OR GREEN)
- ☐ CAULIFLOWER
- ☐ BROCCOLI
- ☐ CARROTS
- ☐ CELERY
- ☐ TOMATO
- ☐ BEET
- ☐ FENNEL RINGS
- ☐ RED ONION
- ☐ AVOCADO
- ☐ SAUERKRAUT
- ☐ NUTRITIONAL YEAST
- ☐ BLUEBERRIES
- ☐ STRAWBERRIES
- ☐ RASPBERRIES
- ☐ BLACKBERRIES
- ☐ CHIA SEEDS
- ☐ FLAX SEEDS
- ☐ HEMP SEEDS
- ☐ WALNUTS
- ☐ PISTACHIOS
- ☐ CASHEWS
- ☐ ALMONDS
- ☐ PECANS
- ☐ MINT
- ☐ BASIL
- ☐ OREGANO
- ☐ DILL
- ☐ FENNEL FRONDS
- ☐ OLIVE OIL
- ☐ APPLE CIDER VINEGAR
- ☐ LEMON

BUILD YOUR BOWL

- ☐ COOKED CUBED SWEET POTATO
- ☐ COOKED BLACK BEANS
- ☐ CUBED AVOCADO
- ☐ ARUGULA
- ☐ WATERCRESS
- ☐ KALE
- ☐ ROMAINE
- ☐ COOKED BULGUR
- ☐ COOKED QUINOA
- ☐ CAULIFLOWER RICE
- ☐ SAUERKRAUT
- ☐ SHREDDED RED OR GREEN CABBAGE
- ☐ CHIA SEEDS
- ☐ FLAX SEEDS
- ☐ HEMP SEEDS
- ☐ SUNFLOWER SEEDS
- ☐ WALNUTS
- ☐ CASHEWS
- ☐ ALMONDS
- ☐ PEPITAS
- ☐ COOKED SALMON
- ☐ TUNA
- ☐ CUBED COOKED TOFU

YOUR BRAIN & YOUR HEART

The vascular component of brain health is very important. Circulation is key for both the heart and the brain.

Your brain and your heart are both at their best with blood pumping to them.

Your brain benefits by managing:

- Diabetes
- High blood pressure
- High cholesterol

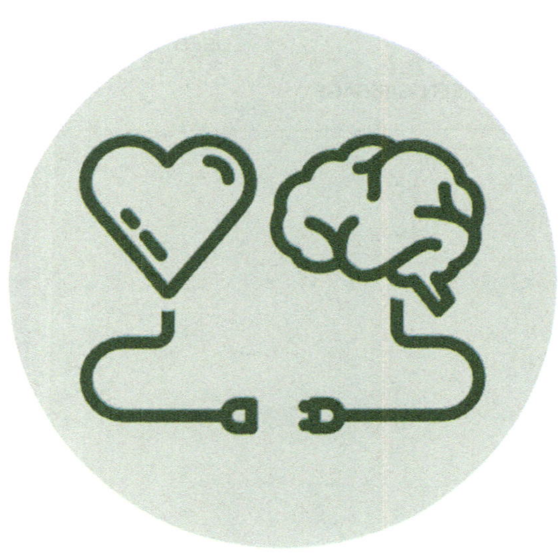

THOUGHTS

Stressful thoughts create hormones that impact body processes.

Chronic high stress creates high levels of cortisol.

Cortisol affects the hippocampus, which is where memories are stored.

Stress can contribute to memory loss and suppresses the immune system.

Manage stress through meditation, mindfulness, breathwork and journaling.

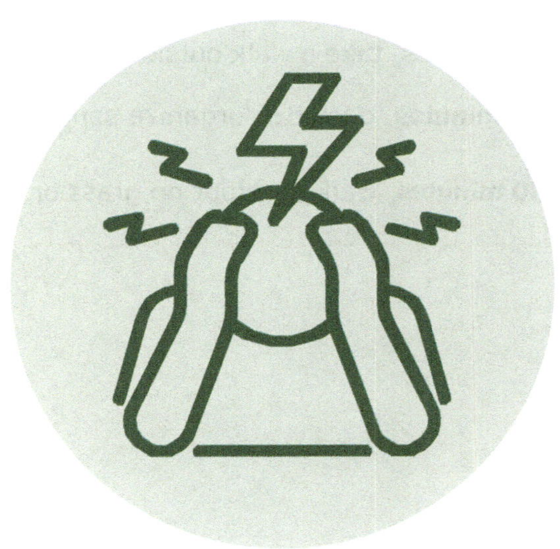

STRESS MANAGEMENT ACTIVITIES

CALM AND FOCUS YOUR MIND

- ☐ If you have **1 minute**, focus and name
  - 5 things you can see,
  - 4 things you can touch
  - 3 things you can hear
  - 2 things you can smell
  - 1 thing you can taste
- ☐ If you have **5 minutes**, sit quietly and focus on only hearing birdsong
- ☐ If you have **10 minutes**, take a walk outside
- ☐ If you have **20 minutes**, declutter/organize something
- ☐ If you have **30 minutes**, walk barefoot on grass or sand

EXERCISE

Your brain needs oxygen.

Exercise produces BDNF (brain derived neurotrophic factor) which is like Miracle Grow for your brain.

Exercise can boost mood and reduce stress.

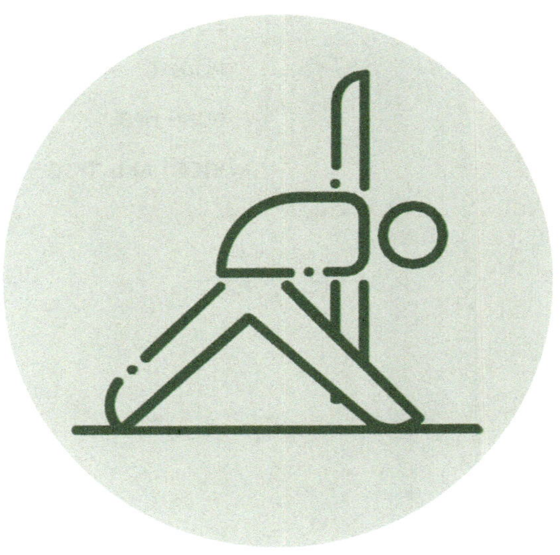

BUILD YOUR BODY

ACTIVITIES TO ADD TO YOUR ROUTINE

BALANCE

- ☐ SINGLE LEG STAND
- ☐ TOE RAISES
- ☐ TAI CHI
- ☐ YOGA

MOBILITY

- ☐ ANKLE CIRCLES
- ☐ LEG SWINGS (FROM STANDING)
- ☐ ARM CIRCLES
- ☐ CAT/ COW

CARDIO

- ☐ WALKING UPHILL
- ☐ STAIR CLIMBING
- ☐ JUMPING ROPE
- ☐ DANCING

STRENGTH

- ☐ SQUATS
- ☐ PLANKS
- ☐ PUSH UPS
- ☐ BICEP AND TRICEP CURLS

YOUR EXERCISE GOALS

TODAY

☐ ______________________________

☐ ______________________________

☐ ______________________________

☐ ______________________________

THIS MONTH

☐ ______________________________

☐ ______________________________

☐ ______________________________

☐ ______________________________

THIS YEAR

☐ ______________________________

☐ ______________________________

☐ ______________________________

☐ ______________________________

EXERCISE TIPS

IDEAS
☐ Habit stack exercise
☐ Keep a tennis ball near bathroom sink, roll out your feet while brushing your teeth
☐ Work on balance while making coffee - stand on one foot for the prep time, the other foot for the brew time
☐ Become an urban hiker. Walk to your errands wearing a backpack for pickups and dropoffs
☐ Keep dumbbells by your bedroom door so every time you walk in or out, you do 10 bicep curls
☐ Set walking dates with friends
☐ Play memory games while on walks with friends
☐ Bring disposable gloves and a plastic bag and pick up litter while walking – bending over moves more muscles
☐ Walk for 10 minutes after every meal, helps regulate blood sugar

SLEEP

Your brain has 85 billion brain cells that create every physiological process in your body.

These cells are like 85 billion factories — busy, busy, busy, all day.

And like a busy factory, at the end of the day, there is garbage that needs to be removed.

Your glymphatic system is at work during deep sleep. This is like a dishwasher or a garbage pickup for debris.

SLEEP

Maximize your sleep environment

- Keep room dark
- Keep room cool
- Minimize screen time prior to bed
- Sleep on your side
- Slow down your nervous system with 4-7-8 breathing technique — breathe in to a count of 4, hold for a count of 7, and exhale for a count of 8

SLEEP TIPS

- ☐ Stop eating 3 hours before bedtime
- ☐ Take an Epsom salt bath
- ☐ Cool down your bedroom
- ☐ Use a sleep eye mask

CONNECTION

The CDC cites that social isolation is associated with about a 50% increased risk of dementia.

25% of adults over 65 are considered to be "socially isolated" — living alone, have had loss of family or friends, have chronic illness, or have hearing loss that isolates them.

Social situations stimulate our brains and engage our neural networks.

CONNECTION

TIPS TO KEEP CONNECTING

- ☐ Schedule time daily to STAY IN TOUCH with family, friends, and neighbors.
  - Not every single person every single day, but at LEAST one person every day.
  - You can call, text or email or visit.
- ☐ Join a book club
- ☐ Organize a potluck on your street
- ☐ Celebrate every occasion
- ☐ Take a class — try pottery, knitting, archery, writing...
- ☐ Join a walking group

CURIOSITY

We all need to have cognitive reserve.

Keep your mind active and never stop learning.

Your brain takes in information like a squirrel hiding nuts.

So, hide the nuts in as many places as you can — read the information, say it, listen to it on audio, and picture it.

Things to keep your brain active

- Playing an instrument
- Learning a language
- Artistic hobby
- Puzzles — pictures or words
- Card games

CURIOSITY

CURIOSITY TIPS

IDEAS

☐ Play a new game

☐ Play cards

☐ Wordle/Connections/Spelling Bee/Strands — challenge yourself to do all 4 (free version of Spelling Bee) in under 20 minutes to start

- When you conquer that, try completing them all in less than 10 minutes

TOXINS

Remember: To support your mitochondria (energy powerhouses that run your
cells), reduce exposure to what damages them (toxins).

Here is a list of Things That Drain Your Brain:

- Exposure to Everyday Toxins:
- Air pollution
- Water
- Treated fabrics/materials in clothing
- Ultra-processed food
- Fragranced products
- Digital content
- Skincare/cosmetics/perfumes
- Cleaning supplies
- Plastic cooking items (cutting boards, utensils that get heated)
- Upholstery off gases (new car smell)

TOXINS

Behaviors that Drain Your Brain:

- Smoking
- Alcohol
- Unaddressed sight or hearing loss
- Unaddressed infection — especially oral
- Unaddressed high blood pressure
- Unaddressed diabetes
- Lack of quality sleep
- Not wearing seat belts or bike helmets

We can't control everything, but we can take an active role in managing many things.

YOU CAN LIMIT YOUR TOXIC LOAD

- Small changes can have big impacts
- Progress, not perfection
- Every little thing matters
- Paying attention pays off

ALCOHOL

Alcohol... to drink or not to drink. That is the question.

And the answer is...
ALCOHOL IS A NEUROTOXIN
Plain and simple.

It's a risk assessment, and then a risk management decision.

Here are some strategies to cut back if you are considering an alcohol-free lifestyle.

- Always have food with alcohol
- Alternate each drink with a glass of water
- Choose organic/clean tequila or wine
- Use lots of ice in drinks, even wine
- Start making delicious mocktails

ALCOHOL

It can be challenging to cut back completely at the outset of your journey.

If you are accustomed to daily cocktails, you can look at the calendar month and allot yourself 15 alcohol days, and 15 alcohol-free days.

Mark every day of the month either A (alcohol day) or AF (alcohol free). This allows you to SEE and track your progress.

If you are at the middle of the month and already have 13 alcohol days in, then you'll want to go with mocktails more often.

Some people use gold stars on their paper calendars to mark their alcohol-free progress.

This gives you a visual report of how you are doing.

When you experience how good you feel on alcohol free days and the mornings after, you will find it easier to have more and more per month.

EPIGENETICS

WHAT IS EPIGENETICS?

Epigenetics is the study of the ENVIRONMENT (the overlay) of the gene.

- Genetic environment is influenced by the foods we eat, and by our thoughts and the hormones they create.
- We can not control our genes, but we may have some say in managing whether they EXPRESS (turn on) or not.
- Think of gene expression as less similar to an on/off switch, like a light switch, and more like a dimmer switch.

INFLAMMATION

WHAT IS INFLAMMATION?

Inflammation gets a bad rap and can sometimes be a good thing.

ACUTE INFLAMMATION

- Happens in response to an injury and lasts a few days
- White blood cells rush to the injury site as a signal
- Does its job to help your body heal

CHRONIC INFLAMMATION

- Can last for weeks, months, or years
- Can cause quite a bit of collateral damage
- If your body floods a site repeatedly with white blood cells, they can end up attacking nearby healthy organs and tissues
- Is at the root of many chronic health issues:
  - arthritis
  - cardiovascular disease
  - diabetes
  - dementia

WORKSHEETS

BRAIN HEALTH ASSESSMENT

That which is not measured cannot be improved!

	Disappointed	OK	Satisfied	Great
Please rate the quality of **food** in your day to day living. Why?:	☐	☐	☐	☐
Please rate the level of **stress** in your day to day living. Why?:	☐	☐	☐	☐
Please rate the quality of **exercise** in your day to day living Why?:	☐	☐	☐	☐
Please rate the quality of **sleep** in your day to day living. Why?:	☐	☐	☐	☐
Please rate the quality of **connection** in your day to day living. Why?:	☐	☐	☐	☐
Please rate the quality of **daily learning** and **brain engagement**. Why?:	☐	☐	☐	☐

WHAT DID I DO FOR MY BRAIN TODAY?

FOOD

- ☐ ______________________________
- ☐ ______________________________
- ☐ ______________________________

STRESS MANAGEMENT

- ☐ ______________________________
- ☐ ______________________________
- ☐ ______________________________

SLEEP

- ☐ ______________________________
- ☐ ______________________________
- ☐ ______________________________

EXERCISE

- ☐ ______________________________
- ☐ ______________________________
- ☐ ______________________________

WHAT DID I DO FOR MY BRAIN TODAY?

BRAIN ENGAGEMENT & LEARNING

- [ ] ______________________
- [ ] ______________________
- [ ] ______________________

CONNECTION/COMMUNITY

- [ ] ______________________
- [ ] ______________________
- [ ] ______________________

THOUGHTS ABOUT THE DAY

____

____

____

____

____

____

____

____

____

____

WHAT DID I DO FOR MY BRAIN TODAY?

FOOD

☐ ____________________
☐ ____________________
☐ ____________________

STRESS MANAGEMENT

☐ ____________________
☐ ____________________
☐ ____________________

SLEEP

☐ ____________________
☐ ____________________
☐ ____________________

EXERCISE

☐ ____________________
☐ ____________________
☐ ____________________

WHAT DID I DO FOR MY BRAIN TODAY?

BRAIN ENGAGEMENT & LEARNING

- ☐ ____________________
- ☐ ____________________
- ☐ ____________________

CONNECTION/COMMUNITY

- ☐ ____________________
- ☐ ____________________
- ☐ ____________________

THOUGHTS ABOUT THE DAY

WHAT DID I DO FOR MY BRAIN TODAY?

FOOD

- ☐ ______________________________
- ☐ ______________________________
- ☐ ______________________________

STRESS MANAGEMENT

- ☐ ______________________________
- ☐ ______________________________
- ☐ ______________________________

SLEEP

- ☐ ______________________________
- ☐ ______________________________
- ☐ ______________________________

EXERCISE

- ☐ ______________________________
- ☐ ______________________________
- ☐ ______________________________

WHAT DID I DO FOR MY BRAIN TODAY?

BRAIN ENGAGEMENT & LEARNING

- ☐ ______________________________
- ☐ ______________________________
- ☐ ______________________________

CONNECTION/COMMUNITY

- ☐ ______________________________
- ☐ ______________________________
- ☐ ______________________________

THOUGHTS ABOUT THE DAY

____

____

____

____

____

____

____

____

____

____

TINY 1%CHANGES

- Drink a glass of water as soon as you wake up
- Stretch before you get out of bed - roll wrists and ankles
- Add cinnamon to your coffee
- Eat an apple every day
- Take a vitamin D capsule
- Do a wall sit for 30 seconds
- Turn the thermostat down in your room at night
- Read/listen to 10 pages of a book
- Listen to a short podcast
- Add one ingredient to your salad
- Add one ingredient to your smoothie
- Add one new herb or spice to anything you are eating
- Get up every hour and walk for 5 minutes
- Walk for 10 minutes after every meal

TINY 1%CHANGES

- Do 10 calf raises while brushing your teeth
- Say thank you 7 times as soon as you open your eyes
- Set ONE intention for the day first thing in the morning
- Replace one topical skin product with a cleaner one
- Get clean laundry detergent when your current brand runs out
- Replace one plastic item in your kitchen with a glass one
- Take away one snack with ingredients that aren't real food
- Drink one less alcoholic drink
- Try riced cauliflower instead of rice
- Add an avocado to your salad
- Eat nuts instead of chips
- Take 4 deep inhales/exhales
- Take a 5 second space before responding to something unpleasant

HABIT STACKING

What can I habit stack?

EXAMPLES OF HABIT STACKING

- ☐ Every day I brush my teeth......I can keep a tennis ball under the sink and roll out my feet while brushing.
- ☐ Every day I make coffee...I can do 12 calf raises while it brews.
- ☐ Every day I gather and toss in a load of laundry...I can listen to 10 minutes of an audio book while I do this.

Every day I ______________________________

I can ______________________________

Every day I ______________________________

I can ______________________________

Every day I ______________________________

I can ______________________________

Every day I ______________________________

I can ______________________________

HABIT STACKING

What can I habit stack?

EXAMPLES OF HABIT STACKING
☐ Every day I brush my teeth......I can keep a tennis ball under the sink and roll out my feet while brushing. ☐ Every day I make coffee...I can do 12 calf raises while it brews. ☐ Every day I gather and toss in a load of laundry...I can listen to 10 minutes of an audio book while I do this. Every day I ____________________ I can ____________________ Every day I ____________________ I can ____________________ Every day I ____________________ I can ____________________ Every day I ____________________ I can ____________________

HABIT STACKING

What can I habit stack?

EXAMPLES OF HABIT STACKING

- ☐ Every day I brush my teeth......I can keep a tennis ball under the sink and roll out my feet while brushing.
- ☐ Every day I make coffee...I can do 12 calf raises while it brews.
- ☐ Every day I gather and toss in a load of laundry...I can listen to 10 minutes of an audio book while I do this.

Every day I ______________________________

I can ______________________________

Every day I ______________________________

I can ______________________________

Every day I ______________________________

I can ______________________________

Every day I ______________________________

I can ______________________________

MAXIMIZE/OPTIMIZE

How can I maximize/optimize?

EXAMPLES MAXIMIZE/OPTIMIZE
☐ I already eat yogurt.....I can add collagen powder ☐ I already eat salad...I can add nutritional yeast ☐ I already made guacamole....I can add chopped pistachios & hemp seeds. I already ____________________ I can ____________________ I already ____________________ I can ____________________ I already ____________________ I can ____________________

MAXIMIZE/OPTIMIZE

How can I maximize/optimize?

EXAMPLES MAXIMIZE/OPTIMIZE

- ☐ I already eat yogurt.....I can add collagen powder
- ☐ I already eat salad...I can add nutritional yeast
- ☐ I already made guacamole....I can add chopped pistachios & hemp seeds.

I already ______________________________

I can ______________________________

I already ______________________________

I can ______________________________

I already ______________________________

I can ______________________________

MAXIMIZE/OPTIMIZE

How can I maximize/optimize?

EXAMPLES MAXIMIZE/OPTIMIZE

- ☐ I already eat yogurt.....I can add collagen powder
- ☐ I already eat salad...I can add nutritional yeast
- ☐ I already made guacamole....I can add chopped pistachios & hemp seeds.

I already ______________________________

I can ______________________________

I already ______________________________

I can ______________________________

I already ______________________________

I can ______________________________

HABIT TRACKING

Keeping track of your habits can help you stay on track and achieve your goals. Fill out your top 12 goals and mark them off each day you successfully complete them.

Habit/Brain Care Step	S	M	T	W	T	F	S
01	☐	☐	☐	☐	☐	☐	☐
02	☐	☐	☐	☐	☐	☐	☐
03	☐	☐	☐	☐	☐	☐	☐
04	☐	☐	☐	☐	☐	☐	☐
05	☐	☐	☐	☐	☐	☐	☐
06	☐	☐	☐	☐	☐	☐	☐
07	☐	☐	☐	☐	☐	☐	☐
08	☐	☐	☐	☐	☐	☐	☐
09	☐	☐	☐	☐	☐	☐	☐
10	☐	☐	☐	☐	☐	☐	☐
11	☐	☐	☐	☐	☐	☐	☐
12	☐	☐	☐	☐	☐	☐	☐

REFLECTION NOTES:

HABIT TRACKING

Keeping track of your habits can help you stay on track and achieve your goals. Fill out your top 12 goals and mark them off each day you successfully complete them.

Habit/Brain Care Step	S	M	T	W	T	F	S
01	☐	☐	☐	☐	☐	☐	☐
02	☐	☐	☐	☐	☐	☐	☐
03	☐	☐	☐	☐	☐	☐	☐
04	☐	☐	☐	☐	☐	☐	☐
05	☐	☐	☐	☐	☐	☐	☐
06	☐	☐	☐	☐	☐	☐	☐
07	☐	☐	☐	☐	☐	☐	☐
08	☐	☐	☐	☐	☐	☐	☐
09	☐	☐	☐	☐	☐	☐	☐
10	☐	☐	☐	☐	☐	☐	☐
11	☐	☐	☐	☐	☐	☐	☐
12	☐	☐	☐	☐	☐	☐	☐

REFLECTION NOTES:

____

____

____

HABIT TRACKING

Keeping track of your habits can help you stay on track and achieve your goals. Fill out your top 12 goals and mark them off each day you successfully complete them.

Habit/Brain Care Step	S	M	T	W	T	F	S
01	☐	☐	☐	☐	☐	☐	☐
02	☐	☐	☐	☐	☐	☐	☐
03	☐	☐	☐	☐	☐	☐	☐
04	☐	☐	☐	☐	☐	☐	☐
05	☐	☐	☐	☐	☐	☐	☐
06	☐	☐	☐	☐	☐	☐	☐
07	☐	☐	☐	☐	☐	☐	☐
08	☐	☐	☐	☐	☐	☐	☐
09	☐	☐	☐	☐	☐	☐	☐
10	☐	☐	☐	☐	☐	☐	☐
11	☐	☐	☐	☐	☐	☐	☐
12	☐	☐	☐	☐	☐	☐	☐

REFLECTION NOTES:

TROUBLESHOOT

For each of the categories below, write down things you are doing well and where you need improvement. Take the time to reflect on these and write a goal for each category.

CATEGORY	WHAT I'M DOING WELL	WHERE I NEED IMPROVEMENT	MY GOALS
FOOD			
STRESS MANAGEMENT			
EXERCISE			
SLEEP			
CONNECTION			
CURIOSITY			

TROUBLESHOOT

For each of the categories below, write down things you are doing well and where you need improvement. Take the time to reflect on these and write a goal for each category.

CATEGORY	WHAT I'M DOING WELL	WHERE I NEED IMPROVEMENT	MY GOALS
FOOD			
STRESS MANAGEMENT			
EXERCISE			
SLEEP			
CONNECTION			
CURIOSITY			

TROUBLESHOOT

For each of the categories below, write down things you are doing well and where you need improvement. Take the time to reflect on these and write a goal for each category.

CATEGORY	WHAT I'M DOING WELL	WHERE I NEED IMPROVEMENT	MY GOALS
FOOD			
STRESS MANAGEMENT			
EXERCISE			
SLEEP			
CONNECTION			
CURIOSITY			

START SMALL

GOAL:

SMALL STEP:

GOAL:

SMALL STEP:

GOAL:

SMALL STEP:

GOAL:

SMALL STEP:

START SMALL

GOAL:

SMALL STEP:

GOAL:

SMALL STEP:

GOAL:

SMALL STEP:

GOAL:

SMALL STEP:

START SMALL

GOAL:

SMALL STEP:

GOAL:

SMALL STEP:

GOAL:

SMALL STEP:

GOAL:

SMALL STEP:

DAILY JOURNAL

HOW DID I SUPPORT MY MICROBIOME TODAY?
(List different foods)

HOW DID I HYDRATE MY BODY AND BRAIN TODAY?

HOW DID I SUPPORT MY MITOCHONDRIA TODAY?
(List toxins avoided)

DAILY JOURNAL

HOW DID I SUPPORT MY MICROBIOME TODAY?
(List different foods)

HOW DID I HYDRATE MY BODY AND BRAIN TODAY?

HOW DID I SUPPORT MY MITOCHONDRIA TODAY?
(List toxins avoided)

DAILY JOURNAL

HOW DID I SUPPORT MY MICROBIOME TODAY?
(List different foods)

HOW DID I HYDRATE MY BODY AND BRAIN TODAY?

HOW DID I SUPPORT MY MITOCHONDRIA TODAY?
(List toxins avoided)

Now that you have this understanding of how your brain works and why you want to keep it at its best, you may be ready to do a little bit of a reset.

We know our body's successful approach to a "detox" is through a healthy diet and regular exercise. But what about when it comes to our minds?

Just as our bodies can retain toxins and waste, our minds can hold on to toxic outlooks and attitudes.

Try these Morning Meditation and Evening Journal prompts to give your mind a chance to clear some things out.

The cookbook framework is brain-fueling breakfast, lunch, dinner and dessert recipes — you can pick and choose what you want and don't have to follow the order of the days.

If you prefer to go more plant-based one day and more protein- based another, feel free to move around the meals to your liking.

If you are not a dessert-lover, skip those.

Some of the recipes make quantities for more than one meal, so please don't get overwhelmed by "all of the cooking".

These recipes have been created to help keep your brain in tip- top condition and have been informed by culinary medicine and functional nutrition. They use ingredients that help minimize inflammation and maximize brain function.

For the most success, find foods that are organic, pasture- raised and grass fed to ensure your brain is getting the cleanest, most chemical-free, pesticide-free and additive-free ingredients you can get.

If you eat well, move well, and think well, you can feel refreshed, renewed, and clear.

What helps your body perform at its best NOW can also help your brain perform at its best for years to come.

THE 7-DAY BRAIN RESET

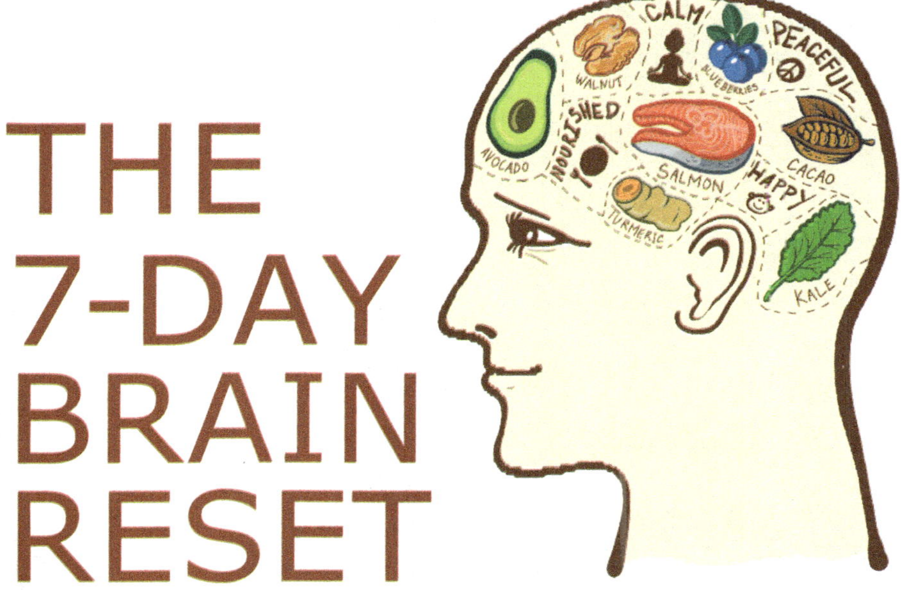

IT'S ALL IN YOUR HEAD

CALM YOUR MIND FEED YOUR BRAIN

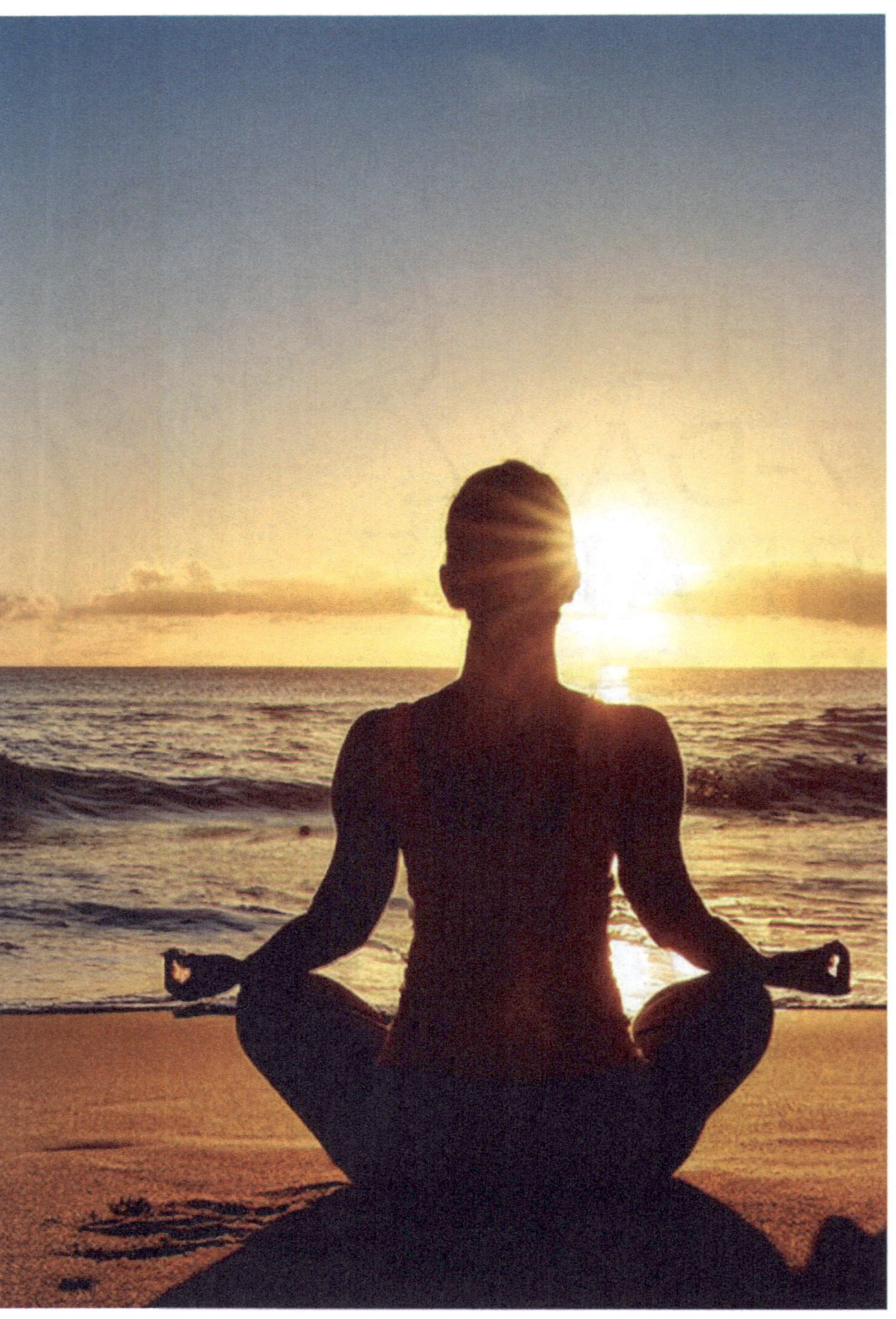

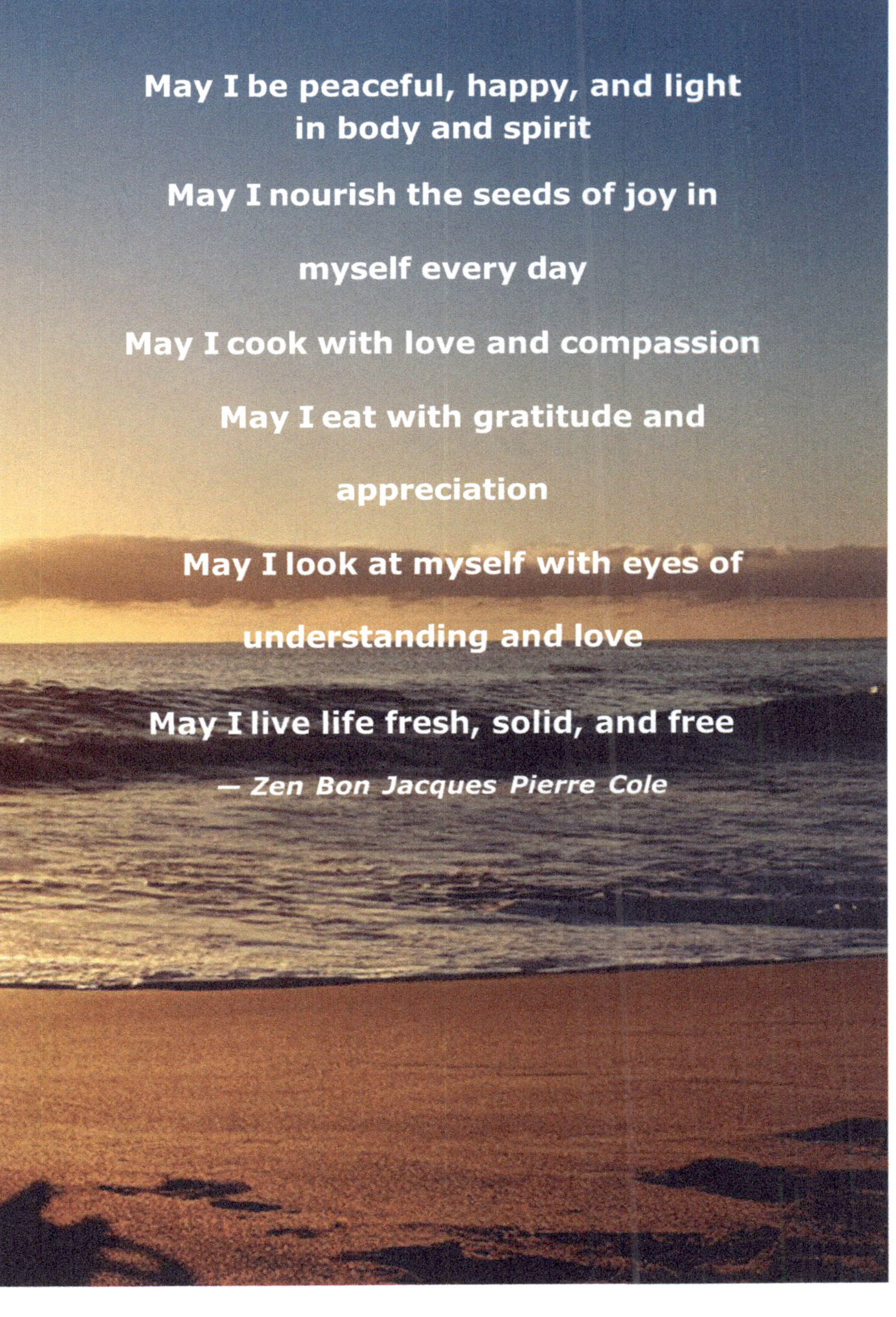
May I be peaceful, happy, and light
in body and spirit
May I nourish the seeds of joy in
myself every day
May I cook with love and compassion
May I eat with gratitude and
appreciation
May I look at myself with eyes of
understanding and love
May I live life fresh, solid, and free
— Zen Bon Jacques Pierre Cole

DAY 1

PRACTICE MINDFULNESS

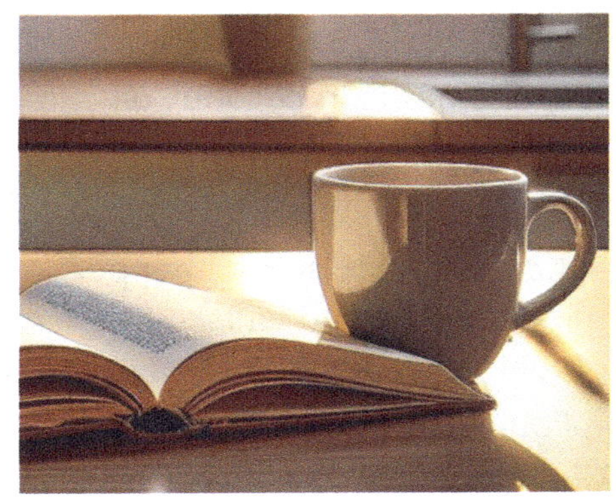

In our everyday life, it is easy for our minds to be influenced by environmental triggers — whether they are stories in the media, advertisements on billboards, or social media posts from friends. Practice becoming aware of those outside influences and analyze the impact they have on your mental state. Today, work to become mindfully present and consider how these influences make you feel.

As you go about your day, stop once in the morning, once in the afternoon, and once before bed (use an alarm on your phone to remind you) to pause and check-in with yourself. Are you stressed, invigorated, overwhelmed?

DAY 1 MENU

BREAKFAST:
Superfood Scramble

Prep time: 5 minutes
Cook time: 5 minutes
Serves: 2-3

INGREDIENTS

- 1 clove garlic, chopped
- 1 tbsp coconut oil
- 4 organic, pasture-raised eggs
- 1/2 tsp turmeric
- 1/4 tsp black pepper
- Sea salt to taste
- 1 tbsp water
- 1/2 cup arugula
- 1/2 an avocado, sliced

STEPS

- Sauté garlic in coconut oil over medium heat
- Break eggs into bowl
- Add water, turmeric, pepper, and sea salt and whisk together
- Pour into skillet with garlic
- Add arugula
- Cook until eggs are at desired consistency
- Top with sliced avocado when plated

Featured Brain Boost Ingredient:
TURMERIC

- Curcumin is a natural anti-inflammatory compound
- Pair with black pepper
- Piperine, a component of black pepper, helps make the anti-inflammatory properties of turmeric more bio-available

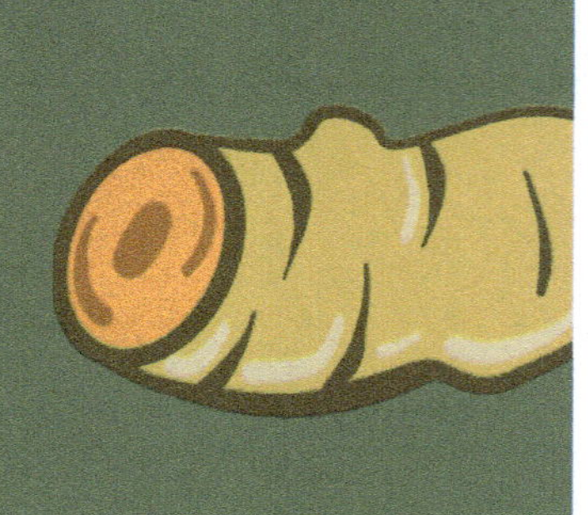

DAY 1 MENU

LUNCH:
Cauliflower Tabbouleh

Prep time: 20 minutes

Cook time: None

Serves: 4

INGREDIENTS

- 3 Persian cucumbers, small dice
- 1 onion, small dice
- 3-4 small tomatoes, small dice (drain excess juice)
- 2 bunches parsley, finely chopped (about 2 cups)
- 1 bunch mint, chopped (about 3/4 cup)
- 2 garlic cloves, small mince
- 1 large cauliflower, rough chopped and riced in food processor
- 3 tbsp olive oil
- 2 tbsp lemon juice

STEPS

- Mix all ingredients in a large bowl

DAY 1 MENU

DINNER:
Roast Lemon Chicken and Oven Roasted Vegetables with Caramelized Garlic

Prep time: 20 minutes

Cook time: 60-90 minutes

Serves: 4

ROASTED CHICKEN

INGREDIENTS

- 1organic, hormone-free chicken
- 1lemon, cut in half
- 2 tbsp of salted butter
- Sea salt & cracked black pepper

STEPS

- Preheat oven to 425°
- Put one lemon half in chicken cavity
- Rub 1tablespoon of butter all over outside of chicken
- Sprinkle salt and pepper over outside of chicken
- Squeeze juice of the remaining lemon half over chicken
- Gently lift breast skin and place the remaining butter underneath
- Roast at 425° for 60-90 minutes, depending on size

Note: Chicken is done when juices run clear

OVEN ROASTED VEGETABLES WITH CARAMELIZED GARLIC

INGREDIENTS

- 3 medium sweet potatoes, peeled, and cut into chunks
- 3 carrots chopped on the diagonal
- 1/2 a yellow onion, quartered twice
- 5 cloves of garlic, each cut in half
- 1/2 tsp turmeric
- Sea salt and cracked black pepper

STEPS

- Put vegetables in baking dish and toss with olive oil to coat
- Add spices and toss again to coat evenly
- Roast at 425° along with chicken for about an hour or until garlic caramelizes

DAY 1 MENU

DESSERT:
Almond Flour Cake

Prep time: 15 minutes

Cook time: 35 minutes

Serves: 6

INGREDIENTS

- 1 1/2 cups almond flour
- 1 1/2 tsp baking powder
- 1/8 tsp sea salt
- 1 tbsp lemon juice
- Zest of one lemon
- 1/4 cup honey
- 1/2 cup olive oil
- 2 eggs
- 10 figs, sliced in half

STEPS

- Heat oven to 350°
- Grease 8in round cake pan and line with parchment
- In large bowl, whisk together lemon juice and zest, honey, olive oil, eggs, and salt
- Add almond flour and baking powder to blend
- Pour batter into pan and arrange figs in batter
- Bake for 35 minutes, or until golden

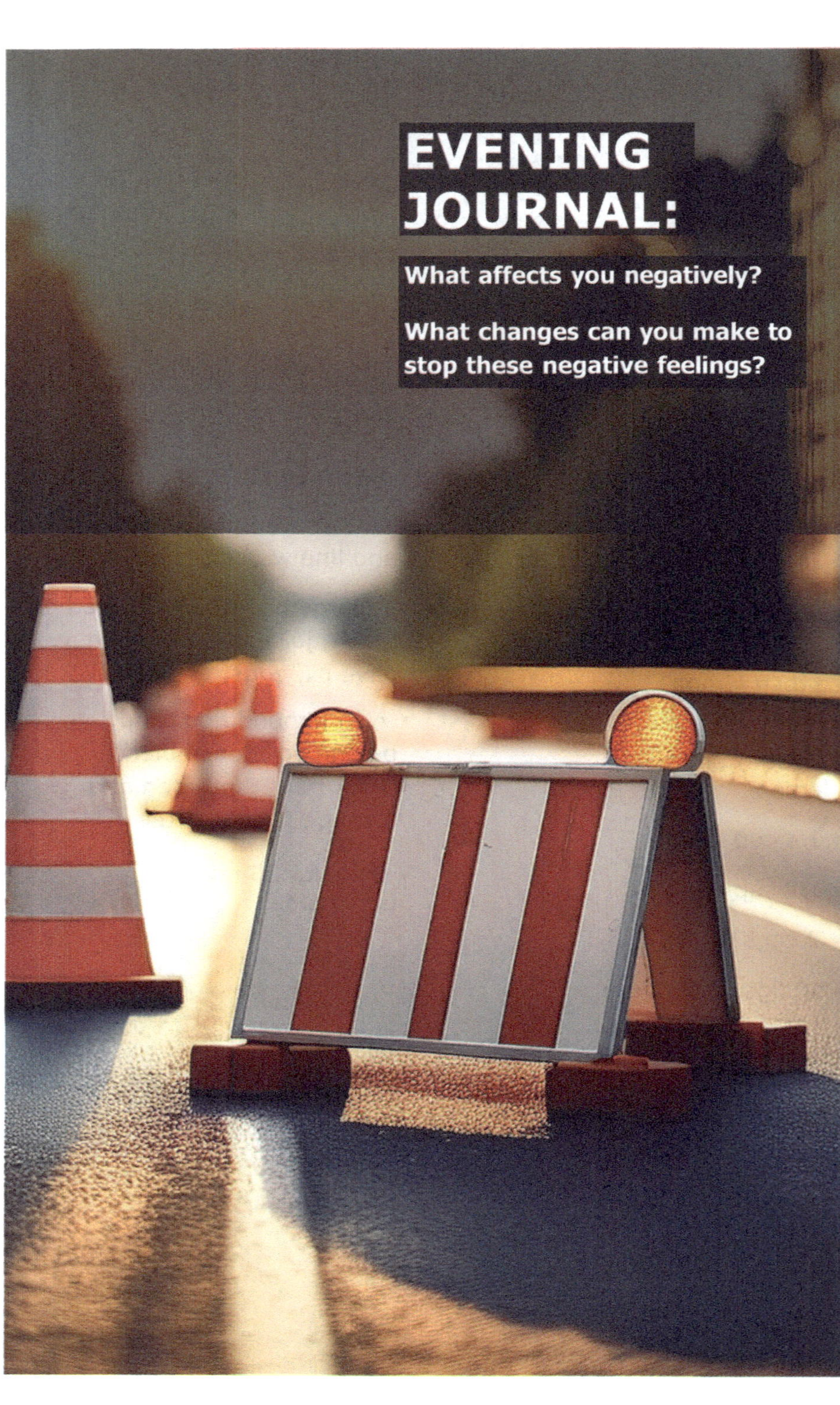
EVENING
JOURNAL:
What affects you negatively?
What changes can you make to stop these negative feelings?

DAY 2

REMOVE THE CHAOS

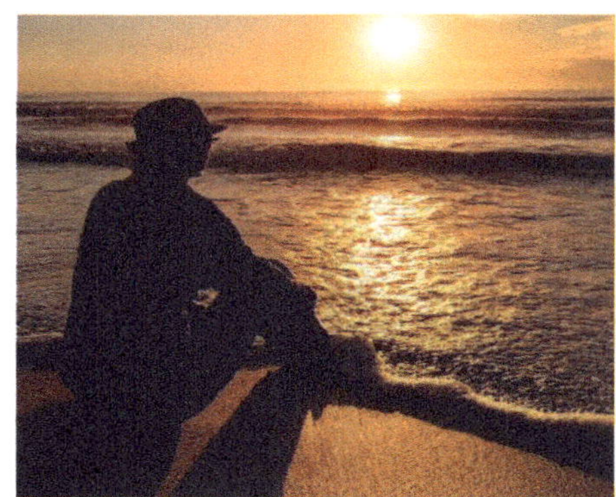

Do you plan your day or week? If not, it can often leave you feeling powerless. Today, mentally organize your day from morning to night. Use a pencil in your schedule and avoid the temptation to fill in every single time slot.

Do your best to stay focused and clear by knowing what you need to be doing when, and actually do it! You won't have to wonder what happened to the day — you will know, and it will lead to increased confidence and security in the days to come.

DAY 2 MENU

BREAKFAST:
Almond Flour Mini Scones

Prep time: 15 minutes

Cook time: 20 minutes

Serves: 6

INGREDIENTS

- 3 cups almond flour
- 1 tsp baking soda
- Dash of salt
- 2 eggs
- 2 tbsp honey
- 1 tbsp fresh lemon or lime juice
- 3 tbsp coconut oil
- 2 tbsp chia seeds

STEPS

- Heat oven to 325°
- Combine almond meal, baking soda, salt, and chia seed
- Add eggs, honey, citrus juice, and coconut oil
- Stir and...
  - Drop by large spoonful onto lightly greased or parchment papered baking sheet
- Bake for 15 - 20 minutes until golden brown

DAY 2 MENU

LUNCH:
Baked Egg with Avocado and Cilantro Lime Sauce

Prep time: 15 minutes

Cook time: 15 minutes

Serves: 2

BAKED EGG WITH AVOCADO

INGREDIENTS

- 1 avocado
- 2 eggs *(size the eggs to your avocado size: Medium avocado to medium eggs or large avocado to large eggs)*
- 1/4 tsp turmeric
- Sea salt and black pepper

STEPS

- Halve avocado and remove pit
- Scoop out avocado (widely, not deeply) about 1 large tbsp avocado for hole where egg will sit
- Carefully crack eggs into bowl, keeping yolks intact. *Note: You could crack egg directly onto avocado, but that can be a little messy/tricky*
- Spoon yolk and white into each avocado half
- Sprinkle with turmeric, salt, and pepper
- Bake at 425° for 12 - 15 minutes
- Drizzle with Cilantro Lime Sauce

CILANTRO LIME SAUCE

INGREDIENTS

- 3/4 cup chopped cilantro
- 1/4 cup lime juice
- 1/2 cup olive oil
- 1 tbsp honey
- Dash of Sea salt to taste

STEPS

- Combine cilantro, lime juice, and honey in blender or small food processor
- Blend on low, pour in olive oil in a steady stream and blend until combined
- Taste test and add salt if needed
- Drizzle over baked avocado halves and serve

Note: Reserve some sauce for Cucumber Radish Salad from Day 3

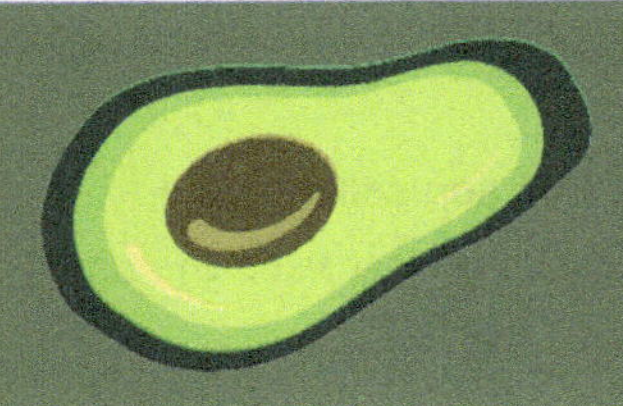

Featured Brain Boost Ingredient:
AVOCADO

- Contains fatty acids that help protect the brain's glial cells
- Fats in avocado are resistant to heat-induced oxidation

DAY 2 MENU

DINNER:
Chicken and Vegetable Soup with Chimichurri Sauce

Prep time: 20 minutes

Cook time: 30 minutes

Serves :4-6

CHICKEN AND VEGETABLE SOUP

INGREDIENTS

- 3 tbsp olive oil
- 1 yellow onion, peeled and diced (about 1 cup)
- 6 cloves garlic, minced
- 2 carrots, peeled and cut crosswise into 1/2-inch pieces
- 2 large or 3 medium celery stalks, cut into 1/2-inch pieces
- 2 bay leaves
- 6 cups chicken broth
- 1 medium zucchini, diced
- 2 (8-ounce) cooked boneless-skinless chicken breast halves, shredded or cut into 1-inch pieces, or leftover pieces from last night's dinner

STEPS

- Heat the olive oil in a stockpot over a medium- high flame
- Add the diced onion, garlic, carrots, and celery and cook until onion is almost translucent, about 3-5 minutes
- Add the bay leaves, 6 cups of broth, and zucchini, and bring to a low simmer
- Cook about 20 minutes or until vegetables are just cooked
- Add shredded chicken breast and heat through
- Remove bay leaf
- When ready ladle into serving bowls and drizzle with Chimichurri sauce right before serving

CHIMICHURRI SAUCE

INGREDIENTS

- 1/4 cup cilantro, roughly chopped
- 3 tbsp lime juice
- 2 teaspoons fresh oregano (if using dried, 1 teaspoon)
- 3 garlic cloves, roughly chopped
- 2 tsp chili flakes
- 1/2 cup olive oil
- Dash of salt

STEPS

- Combine the first six ingredients in a blender or food processor and pulse until combined Don't totally puree as it is good to still have some texture to the sauce
- Test taste and add salt to taste

Note: This sauce is best used the day made

DAY 2 MENU

DESSERT:
Chocolate Chip Cookies

Prep time: 15 minutes

Cook time: 13 minutes

Serves: 4-6

INGREDIENTS

- 2 cups almond flour
- 1/4 tsp baking soda
- 1/4 tsp sea salt
- 1 egg
- 1/4 cup coconut oil, melted and cooled
- 1/4 cup maple syrup
- 1/2 cup chocolate chips

STEPS

- Heat oven to 350°
- Mix flour, baking soda, and salt
- Fold in egg, coconut oil, and maple syrup

  Use measuring cup for maple syrup that you just used for coconut oil, and it slides out easily
- Fold in chocolate chips
- Drop by rounded teaspoons onto parchment- lined cookie sheet
- Bake at 350° for 13 minutes, until golden brown around the edges
- Let cool for ~10 minutes and then enjoy!

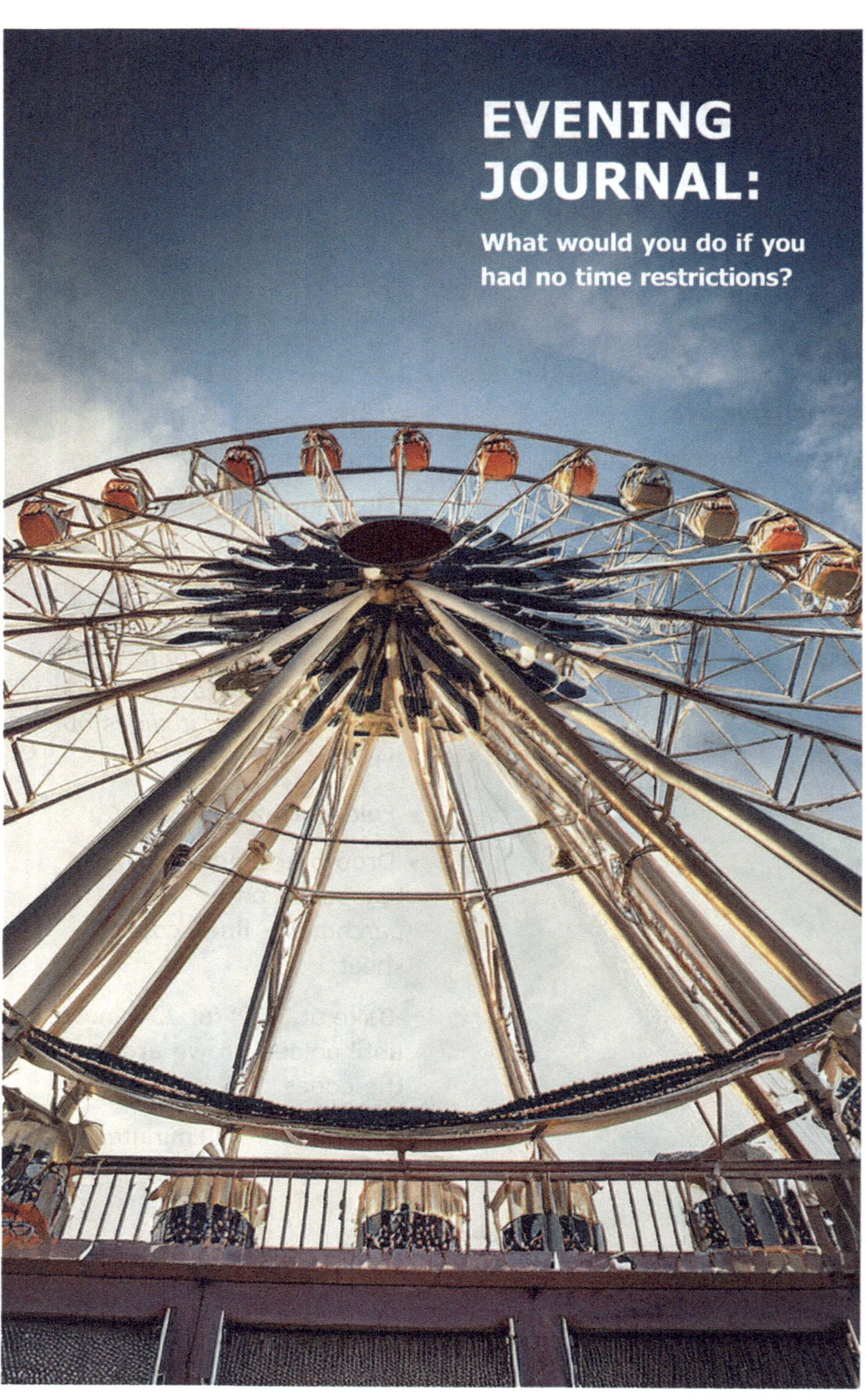
EVENING
JOURNAL:
What would you do if you
had no time restrictions?

DAY 3
LET GO

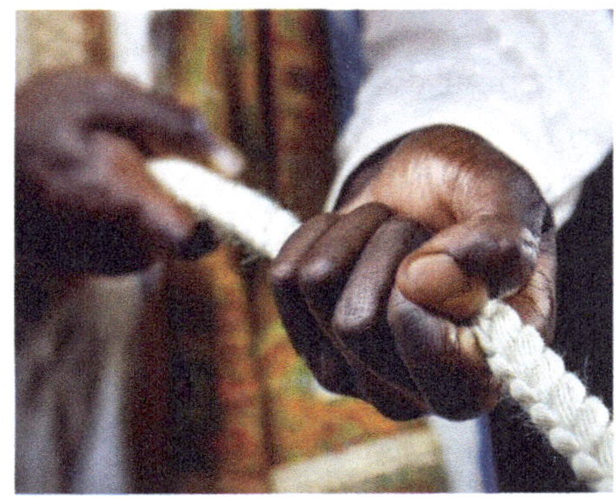

"I don't have enough time" and "I have so much going on" – you probably hear phrases like this daily. Maybe you even say them yourself. People can often list their never- ending montage of tasks verbatim and end with a flurry of "Whew!"

They're obsessed with handling every one of life's details and they love the feeling of control. This can create a mountain of stress. It's time for you to look at yourself and your to-do list. Is it creating stress for you?
Time to let things go. Today, look for ways to delegate your energy to those tasks that are most important and drop the rest.

DAY 3 MENU

BREAKFAST:
Grain-free Granola

Prep time: 15 minutes

Cook time: 20 minutes

Serves: 4

INGREDIENTS

- 1 cup almonds
- 1 cup cashews
- 1/4 cup pumpkin seeds
- 1/4 cup sunflower seeds
- 1/2 cup coconut flakes
- 1/4 cup coconut oil
- 1/2 cup raw honey
- 1 tsp vanilla
- 1 tsp salt

STEPS

- Preheat oven to 275°
- Put nuts/seeds/coconut in processor
- Pulse until you have some coarse grind and some bigger pieces
- Melt coconut oil/honey/vanilla over medium heat
- Add nuts to melted mixture and coat
- Spread out on a baking sheet lined with parchment paper and bake 20 minutes
- When you remove the baking sheet after 20 minutes, add sea salt
- Save some for tomorrow's breakfast yogurt parfait

DAY 3 MENU

LUNCH:
Sweet Potato Kale Soup

Prep time: 30 minutes

Cook time: 1 hour

Serves: 4

INGREDIENTS

- 2 tbsp olive or coconut oil
- 1 red onion, diced
- 2 cloves garlic, minced
- 1 1/2 lbs. sweet potatoes, peeled and cut into chunks
- 6 cups chicken bone broth (or 3 cups plus 3 cups vegetable broth or water)
- 1/4 tsp red pepper flakes
- 1/2 lb. kale leaves, stems removed, and chiffonade cut
- 2 tsp apple cider vinegar

STEPS

- In soup pot, sauté onion and garlic for 5 minutes
- Add sweet potatoes and broth
- Bring to a boil
- Reduce to a simmer and cover
- Simmer 30 minutes
- Remove from heat and mash potatoes roughly – leave some pieces
- Return to low heat, add red pepper and kale, and simmer 30 more minutes
- Stir in vinegar and serve

DAY 3 MENU

DINNER: Ginger Salmon with Mango Mint Salsa and Cucumber Radish Salad

Prep time: 30 minutes

Cook time: 8-10 minutes

Serves: 4

GINGER SALMON

INGREDIENTS

- 4 6 oz salmon fillets
- 3 tbsp minced ginger
- 1 tsp turmeric
- 1 tbsp olive oil
- Dash of sea salt

STEPS

- Preheat oven to 375°
- Mix ginger, turmeric, oil, and salt and rub into salmon
- Heat sauté pan to high heat
- Cook salmon undisturbed, one minute per side. *It will get smoky, be sure to have good ventilation*
- Flip once to get a sear
- Transfer to oven to cook through, around 5 minutes
- Arrange on platter and top with mango mint salsa

Featured Brain Boost Ingredient: **SALMON**

- Contains fatty acids that help protect the brain's glial cells
- Rich source of omega 3 fatty acids
- Contains EPA and DHA
- Excellent source of protein

MANGO MINT SALSA

INGREDIENTS

- 1 mango, medium diced
- 1 jalapeño, seeds discarded, minced
- 1/4 cup red onion, diced
- 1/4 cup of mint leaves, chopped

STEPS

- Combine all ingredients in a mixing bowl and toss gently to combine

CUCUMBER RADISH SALAD WITH CILANTRO LIME DRESSING:

INGREDIENTS

- 1 pound either, or a mix of English, Persian, Japanese cucumber, peeled and sliced on the diagonal
- 1 bunch radishes, trimmed and sliced
- 1/2 cup chopped cilantro

STEPS

- Arrange cucumbers on platter, top with radishes
- Drizzle with Cilantro Lime Sauce, (recipe from Day 2 menu) and garnish with chopped cilantro

DAY 3 MENU

DESSERT:
Berry Trio with Cashew Cream

Advance time: 6 hours
Prep time: 10 minutes
Serves: 4

BERRY TRIO

INGREDIENTS

- Raspberries
- Blueberries
- Blackberries

STEPS

- Wash and drain all berries
- Put berries in a dessert dish
- Top with Cashew Cream

CASHEW CREAM

INGREDIENTS

- 1 cup of cashews
- 1/2 cup water
- 1 tbsp maple syrup
- Dash of sea salt
- A sprig of mint leaves

STEPS

- Soak one cup raw cashews in water for about 6 hours. Drain and rinse the cashews
- Put soaked cashews in food processor with 1/4 cup water
- Process until desired consistency. Add water slowly if mixture is too thick
- Drizzle in 1 tbsp maple syrup and a pinch of sea salt
- Process again and chill
- When ready to serve, remove from refrigerator and top with mint leaves

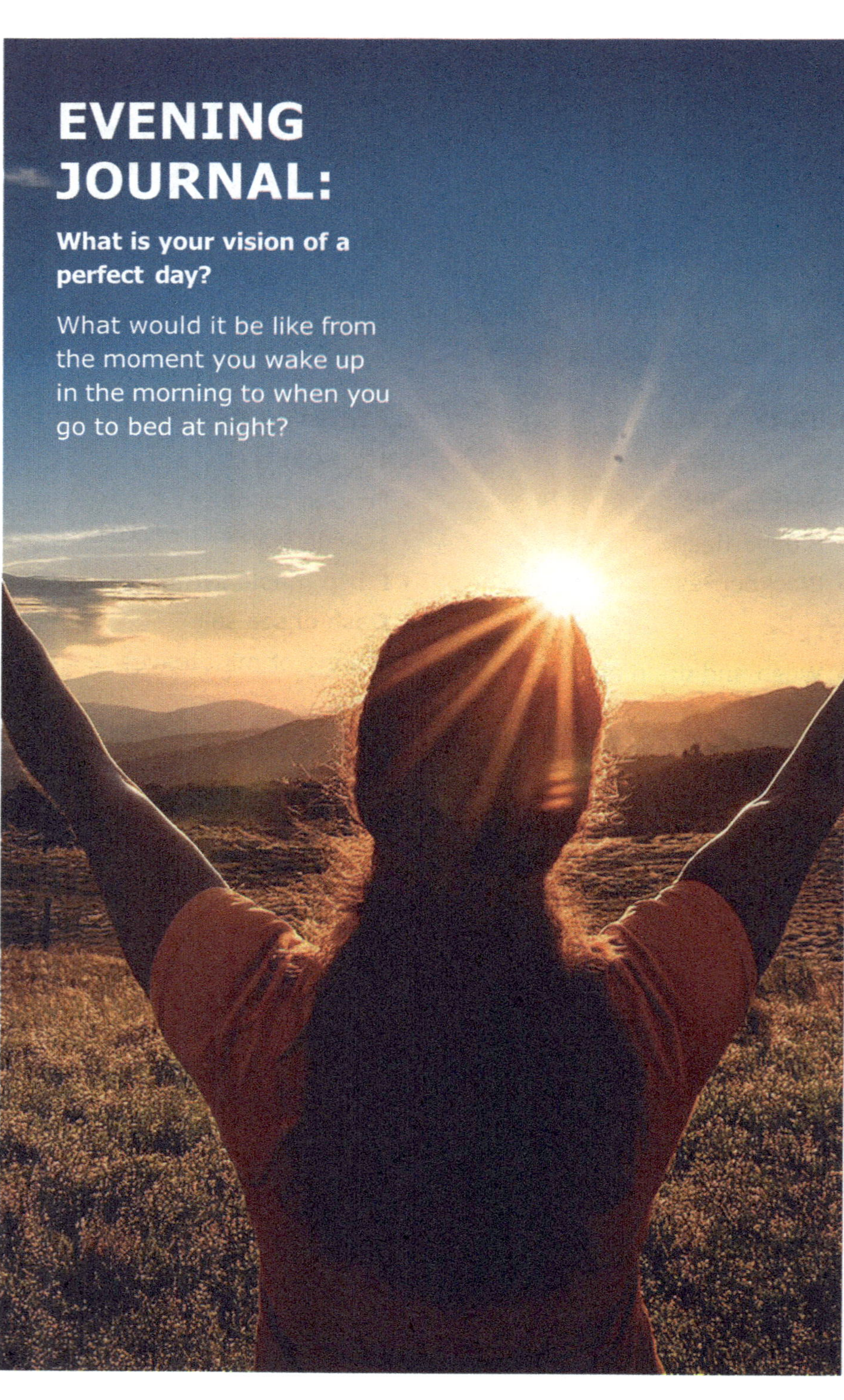
EVENING
JOURNAL:
What is your vision of a perfect day?
What would it be like from the moment you wake up in the morning to when you go to bed at night?

DAY 4

EXPRESS GRATITUDE

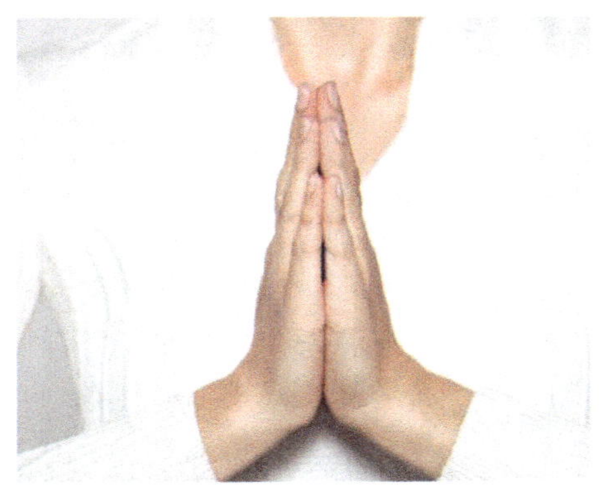

Today, work to harness gratitude. Flip through your phone pictures and let joyous memories wash over you. Write a positive mantra on your bathroom mirror, place sticky notes in random spots.

Do this all throughout your home and leave them up for the week. (Use a dry erase marker for your mirror)

DAY 4 MENU

BREAKFAST:
Yogurt Parfait

Prep time: 5 minutes

Serves: 1

INGREDIENTS

- Organic yogurt
- 1/4 cup grain-free granola you made yesterday
- 1/2 cup blueberries or raspberries or blackberries

STEPS

- In a tall glass or jar that makes you happy, layer organic yogurt with 1/4 cup grain- free granola that you made yesterday
- Add another layer of yogurt and top with fresh blueberries, raspberries, or blackberries

Featured Brain Boost Ingredient:
BLUEBERRIES

- Contains antioxidants that help combat oxidative stress, which can negatively affect brain function

DAY 4 MENU

LUNCH:
Kale Salad with Honey Mustard Vinaigrette

Prep time: 25 minutes

Serves: 4

KALE SALAD:

INGREDIENTS

- 1 bunch green kale stems removed
- 1 bunch red kale, stems removed
- 8 dates, pitted and chopped
- 1/2 cup blueberries
- 1/4 cup chopped honey roasted almonds
- 2 hard-boiled eggs, chopped
- 1 avocado, chopped or sliced

STEPS

- Chiffonade kale
- Place in salad bowl and toss with other ingredients
- Toss in Honey Mustard Vinaigrette

HONEY MUSTARD VINAIGRETTE DRESSING:

INGREDIENTS

- 1/4 cup olive oil
- 2 tbsp Balsamic vinegar
- 1 tbsp honey
- 1 tsp rustic mustard
- 1 tbsp lime juice

STEPS

- Put all ingredients in a glass jar, cover, and shake until well blended
- Pour over Kale Salad and serve

DAY 4 MENU

DINNER:

Shrimp Bites Wrapped in Greens with Minty Cilantro Dressing and Curry Roasted Cauliflower

SHRIMP Prep time: 25 minutes **Cook time:** 6-8 minutes **Serves:** 4
CAULIFLOWER Prep time: 15minutes **Cook time:** 60 minutes **Serves:** 4

SHRIMP BITES

INGREDIENTS

- 6 large shrimp, peeled, de-veined, tails removed
- Olive oil
- 3 collard green leaves, cut into 2-inch squares
- 1/2 cup toasted coconut
- 1/2 cup roasted pepitas
- 2 inches fresh ginger cut into thin matchsticks
- 1 lime sliced very thin
- 2 jalapeno chilis, sliced into thin circles
- Dash of sea salt

STEPS

- Heat grill pan over medium-high or preheat broiler to high
- Lightly coat shrimp with olive oil and season with salt
- Grill shrimp until firm and opaque, about 3 minutes per side
- Split each shrimp into 2 pieces by slicing them down the back
- Lay collard squares flat on a tray
- Place a shrimp half on the collard square
- Top each shrimp half with a sprinkle of toasted coconut, some pepitas, ginger matchsticks, a few rings of chili, lime,
- Drizzle with Minty Cilantro Dressing and serve

MINTY CILANTRO DRESSING

INGREDIENTS

- 1/2 cup cilantro leaves
- 1/2 cup mint leaves
- 1/4 cup olive oil
- 3 tbsp lemon juice
- 1 tsp honey

STEPS

- Combine all ingredients in a blender or processor
- Pulse until combined
- Use immediately or store, covered, in refrigerator, lasts up to 2 days
- Save some for tomorrow's Carrot Ginger Soup

DAY 4 MENU

DINNER – CONTINUED:
Shrimp Bites Wrapped in Greens with Minty Cilantro Dressing and Curry Roasted Cauliflower

Shrimp Prep time: 25 minutes **Cook time:** 6-8 minutes **Serves:** 4
Cauliflower Prep time: 15 minutes **Cook time:** 60 minutes **Serves:** 4

CURRY ROASTED CAULIFLOWER

INGREDIENTS

- 1 head cauliflower (at room temp is easier – coconut oil won't harden on contact) separated into florets — chop any extra stem also
- 1/4 cup melted coconut oil
- 1 tbsp curry powder
- 1 tsp turmeric powder
- 1/2 cup cashews

STEPS

- Preheat the oven to 375°
- Mix oil and powders in a measuring cup
- Put cauliflower in glass baking dish
- Drizzle oil mixture onto cauliflower
- Toss well to coat evenly
- Roast for 45 minutes
- Remove from oven, toss in cashews, cracked pepper, and sea salt
- Mix well and roast 15 more minutes
- Remove and ready to serve

DAY 4 MENU

DESSERT: Sea Salt Coconut Pecan Brownies

Prep time: 10 minutes

Cook time: 20 minutes

Serves: 4-6

INGREDIENTS

- 3/4 cup almond flour
- 5 tbsp cacao powder
- 1/4 tsp baking soda
- 1/2 cup chopped pecans
- 1/2 cup honey
- 2 eggs
- 1/4 cup liquid coconut oil, melted and cooled
- 2 tsp vanilla
- Couple turns of sea salt grinder
- Cacao nibs and toasted coconut for topping

STEPS

- Preheat oven to 325°
- Grease an 8x8 glass baking dish
- Mix all ingredients (except cacao nibs and coconut) in bowl
- Pour mixture into greased baking dish
- Bake for 20 minutes
- Sprinkle with cacao nibs, toasted coconut, and 2 more turns of sea salt grinder

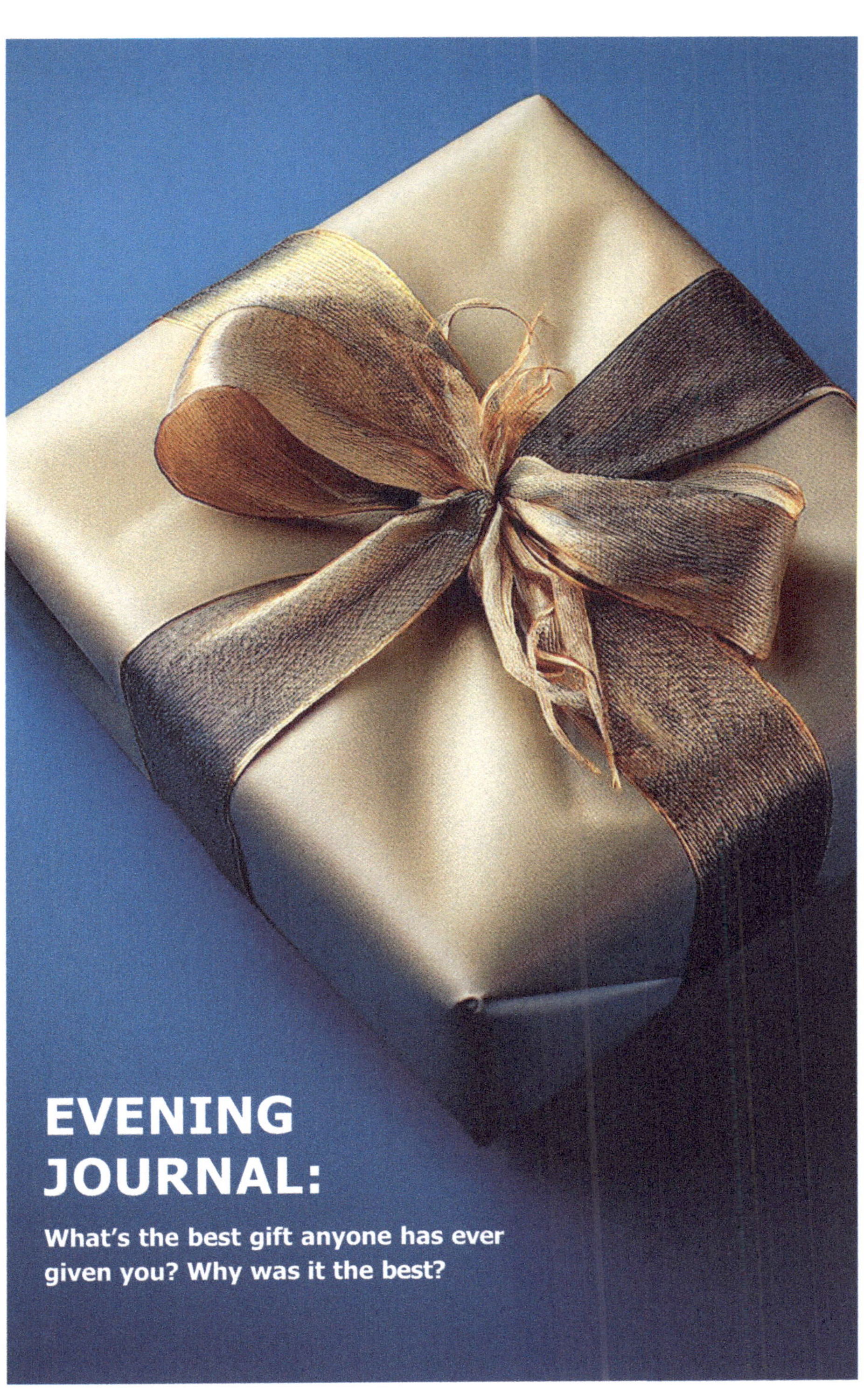

EVENING JOURNAL:

What's the best gift anyone has ever given you? Why was it the best?

DAY 5

TOSS YOUR BROKEN RECORDS

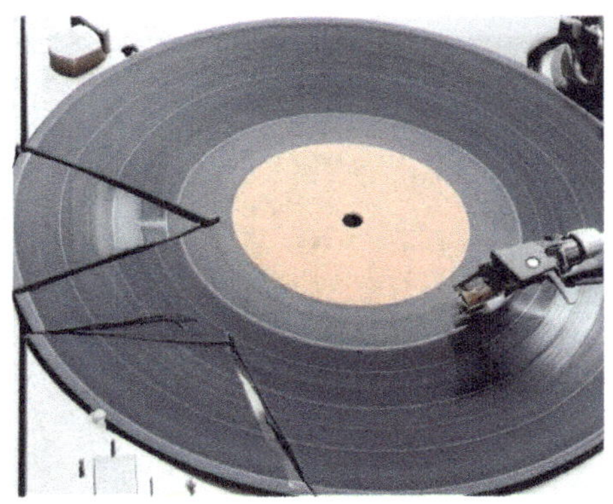

One of the most destructive games our mind plays with itself is replaying painful events on a loop. Someone could have said or done something hurtful to us years ago, and our mind will hit rewind and punch play over and over again.

When those negative thoughts arise today, acknowledge them and throw them away. Choose to focus on the here and now.

DAY 5 MENU

BREAKFAST:

Morning Sunshine Green Drink

Prep time: 10 minutes

Serves: 2

INGREDIENTS

- 3 cups of any combo of: Kale, Arugula, Spinach, or Red/green lettuce
- 1/2 cucumber, cut into chunks
- 1 orange, peeled and seeded
- 1 tbsp seeds — chia, hemp, or flax
- 1 tsp apple cider vinegar
- 1 scoop collagen powder
- 1 scoop beet powder
- 1/4" chunk of peeled ginger (optional)
- Place all ingredients in blender
- Add 2-3 cups icy cold water

STEPS

- Process until smooth

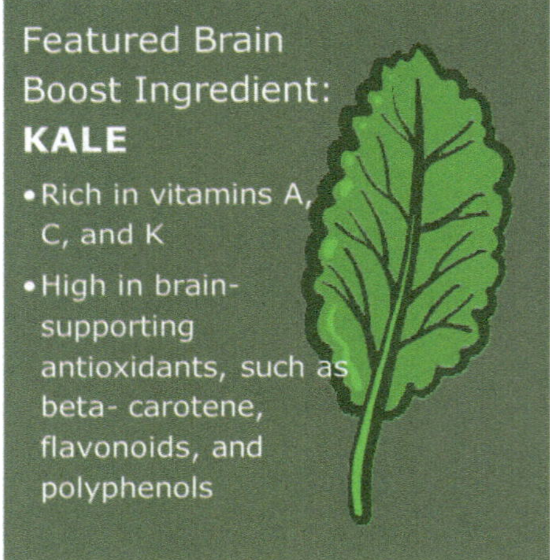

DAY 5 MENU

LUNCH:
Carrot Ginger Soup

Prep time: 15 minutes

Cook time: 40 minutes

Serves: 4

INGREDIENTS

- 3 tbsp olive oil
- 1 yellow onion, diced
- 4 cloves garlic, peeled and chopped
- 5 carrots, diced
- 2 stalks of celery, diced
- 1 tbsp cumin
- 1 tbsp turmeric
- 1/4 cup roughly chopped peeled ginger
- 4 cups vegetable or bone broth, more or less to desired consistency
- Dash of Sea salt

STEPS

- Heat oil over medium in a stockpot
- Add onion and garlic, cook 2 minutes
- Add remaining ingredients, except salt
- Cook over medium heat until vegetables are soft
- Purée with an immersion blender or pour into countertop blender in small batches and purée until smooth
- Season with sea salt
- Swirl in some reserved Minty Cilantro Dressing if desired

DAY 5 MENU

DINNER: 3 Seed Crusted Salmon with Balsamic Braised Cabbage

FISH Prep time: 15 minutes **Cook time:** 10 minutes **Serves:** 4
CABBAGE Prep time: 15 minutes **Cook time:** 45 minutes **Serves:** 4

SALMON

INGREDIENTS

- 4 six-ounce salmon fillets, skin removed
- 1/2 cup lightly pan toasted black sesame seeds
- 1/2 cup lightly pan toasted pepitas
- 1/2 cup lightly pan toasted sunflower seeds
- 1 tsp coarse salt
- Olive oil
- 1 avocado, sliced

STEPS

- Heat the oven to 350°
- Pulse seeds and salt in grinder, blender or processor — Don't pulse or process too long, you want some texture, not a powder
- Put ground seed mixture in a shallow dish or bowl
- Rub and coat the fish lightly with some oil
- Dredge each fillet in the ground seed mix Gently press each side of the fish
- Heat 1/8-inch olive oil on medium heat
- Brown fish about 2 minutes each side, then transfer to a 350° oven and bake until opaque — about 5 minutes, depending on thickness
- Arrange salmon on platter, top with sliced avocado

CABBAGE

INGREDIENTS

- One head red cabbage, cored and sliced
- 1/4 onion, chopped
- 1 tbsp coconut oil
- 1 cup water
- 1/2 cup balsamic vinegar
- 1 tbsp honey
- 1 bay leaf
- Sea salt and cracked black pepper

STEPS

- In a large, lidded pan, sauté onion and cabbage in coconut oil until soft
- Add water, vinegar, honey, bay leaf, salt, and pepper
- Cover and simmer on low 45 minutes
- Remove bay leaf

DAY 5 MENU

DESSERT:
No-Bake Coffee Cacao Pie

Prep time: 25 minutes

Freeze time: 2-3 hours

Serves: 6

CRUST

INGREDIENTS

- 2 cups walnuts
- 8 pitted dates
- Coconut oil to grease 9" pie dish/pan
- 1/2 tsp sea salt

STEPS

- Process walnuts and dates in food processor until it's a coarse paste
- Press date and walnut paste into greased (coconut oil) 9" pie dish
- Refrigerate while making filling

FILLING

INGREDIENTS

- 2 large avocados
- 1 cup cacao powder
- 1/2 cup honey
- 1/4 cup brewed, cooled coffee
- 1/4 cup coconut oil, melted and at room temperature
- 1/2 cup almonds (or hazelnuts or pecans) toasted and coarsely chopped
- Large flake sea salt

STEPS

- Put all ingredients except nuts and sea salt into food processor or blender
- Process until creamy
- Spoon filling into chilled pie crust
- Top the pie filling with the chopped nuts and large sea salt flakes
- Put the finished pie into the freezer to set
- Serving options: Enjoy frozen or leave
  the pie out at room temperature for about 15 minutes.

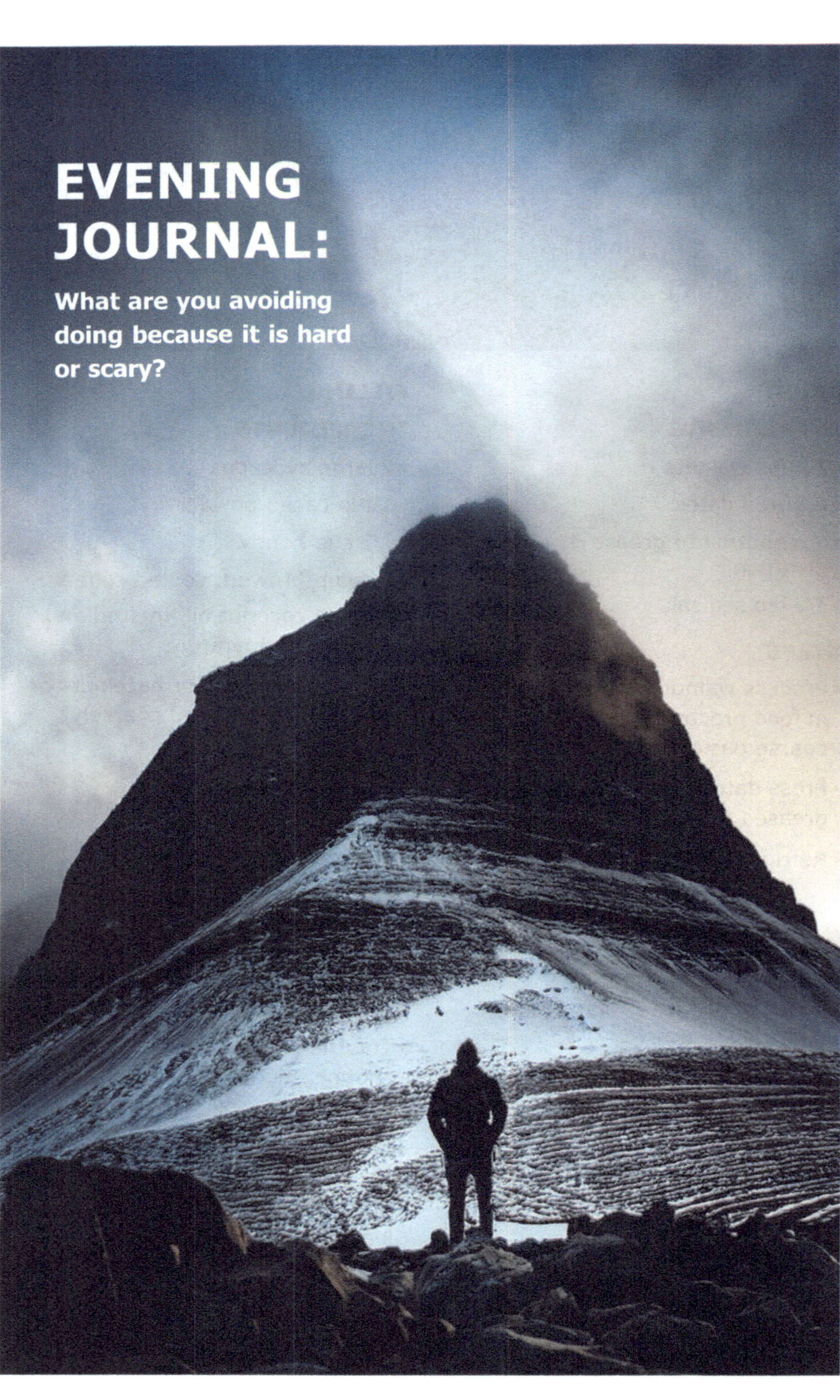
EVENING
JOURNAL:
What are you avoiding
doing because it is hard
or scary?

DAY 6

RESIST BEING REACTIVE

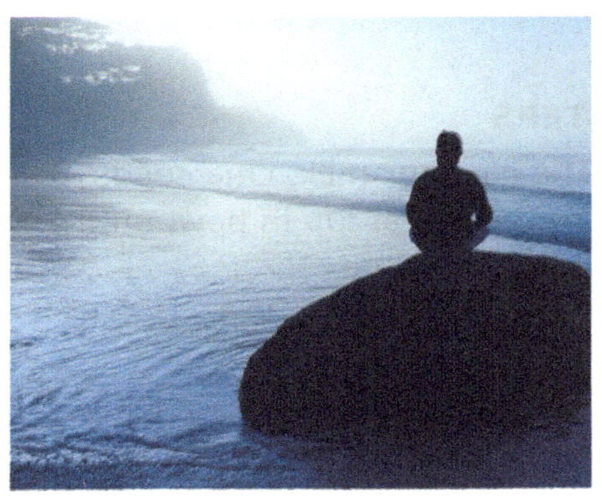

Today, it's time to take a breath and reflect. Maybe even try meditation. Let's reflect on the first five days. Did you respond mindfully to the situations placed in front of you? Are you creating stress by replaying moments in your mind? When did your mind and mouth get out of control?

DAY 6 MENU

BREAKFAST:
Coconut Chia Pudding with Berries

Prep time: 5 minutes

Refrigerator time: 3 hours – overnight

Serves: 4

INGREDIENTS

- 2 cups full fat coconut milk
- 1/2 cup chia seeds
- 2 tbsp agave syrup
- Any berries in season

STEPS

- Mix coconut milk, chia seeds and agave syrup in bowl until fully combined
- Refrigerate mixture at least 3 hours, or best if left overnight
- Remove mixture from refrigerator – it should have a thick pudding-like consistency
- Layer pudding with berries in parfait glasses and serve

DAY 6 MENU

LUNCH:

Carrot Top Pesto Quinoa Bowl

Prep time: 20 minutes

Cook time: 20 minutes

Serves: 2

INGREDIENTS

- 1/2 cup carrot top greens, blanched, tough stems removed
- 1/2 cup arugula or watercress or basil
- 1 large clove garlic, cut in thirds
- 1/4 cup raw cashews
- Sea salt/cracked black pepper
- 1 tbsp olive oil, or a little more if you prefer
- 1 cup cooked quinoa

STEPS

- Put first 5 ingredients into a food processor
- Pulse the mixture and scrape down sides until combined
- Gradually drizzle oil into the food processor while pulsing. Continue to scrape down the sides and pulse the mixture until smooth
- Put quinoa in a large bowl
- Top with mixture from the food processor and gently fold together before serving

DAY 6 MENU

DINNER:
Abundance Brain-Boosting Salad, Rustic Crackers and Cashew Tzatziki

Prep time: 1hour

Cook time: 30 minutes

Serves: 4

ABUNDANCE BRAIN-BOOSTING SALAD

INGREDIENTS

- 5 cups greens, torn into pieces (heavy on arugula)
- 2 avocados
- 1/4 red onion, thinly sliced
- 1/4 cup pistachios, chopped in half
- 1/4 hemp seeds
- 1/4 cup blueberries
- 1/4 cup fresh mint, chopped
- 1/4 cup cilantro, chopped

STEPS

- Toss ingredients in bowl
- Top with dressing

CITRUS MUSTARD TURMERIC DRESSING

INGREDIENTS

- 1/4 cup fresh squeezed lemon or orange juice
- 2 tbsp Dijon mustard
- 1 tbsp Turmeric
- 2 tbsp honey
- 2/3 cup olive oil
- Couple twists of black pepper and sea salt

STEPS

- In a bowl, whisk together juice, mustard, olive oil, turmeric, honey, sea salt and black pepper

DAY 6 MENU

DINNER – CONTINUED:
Abundance Brain-Boosting Salad, Rustic Crackers and Cashew Tzatziki

Prep time: 1hour

Cook time: 30 minutes

Serves: 4

RUSTIC CRACKERS

INGREDIENTS

- 1 1/2 cups almond flour
- 1/2 cup sunflower seeds, some roughly crushed
- Sea salt
- 1 egg
- 1 tbsp olive oil
- 1 tbsp honey
- 1 tbsp chia seeds
- 1 tbsp flax seeds
- 1 tbsp hemp seeds

STEPS

- Mix flour, salt, and seeds
- Whisk egg with oil and add with honey to dry ingredients
- Form a ball
- Roll it out thinly (cracker height) between 2 pieces of parchment
- Bake on bottom parchment on baking sheet 10- 12 minutes (watch closely)
- Break into cracker-sized irregular pieces when cooled

CASHEW TZATZIKI

INGREDIENTS

- 1 1/2 cups cashews, soaked (1 hr in hot water, drain)
- 1 cucumber, peeled and grated
- 2 cloves garlic, minced
- 3/4 tsp sea salt
- 6 tbsp lemon juice
- 2 tbsp white vinegar
- 1/2 -3/4 cup water
- 4 tbsp fresh minced dill
- Cracked black pepper

STEPS

- Blend all but cucumber & dill until smooth and creamy
- Add cucumber & dill

DAY 6 MENU

Dessert: Cacao Bark

Prep time: 10 minutes

Freeze time: 25 minutes - SPLIT

Serves: 4-6

INGREDIENTS

- 1/2 cup melted coconut oil
- 1/3 cup cacao powder
- 1 tsp vanilla
- 1 tsp honey
- 1 tsp chia and/or hemp seeds
- 1 tbsp cashews
- 2 tbsp blueberries
- 2 tsp sunflower seeds
- 2 tsp coconut flakes
- 2 tsp cacao nibs
- Drizzle of honey to top off bark

STEPS

- Melt coconut oil in large bowl
- Mix oil cacao, vanilla and honey in 8x8 baking dish lined with parchment
- Pour in mixture
- Freeze no more than FIVE minutes – the mixture needs to stay soft enough for toppings to stick
- Add toppings
- Freeze 20 minutes more until fully solid
- Break into large pieces
- Store in airtight container in freezer

Featured Brain Boost Ingredient:
CACAO

- Contains flavanols that can reduce inflammation
- Contains phytonutrients that can increase blood flow to the brain

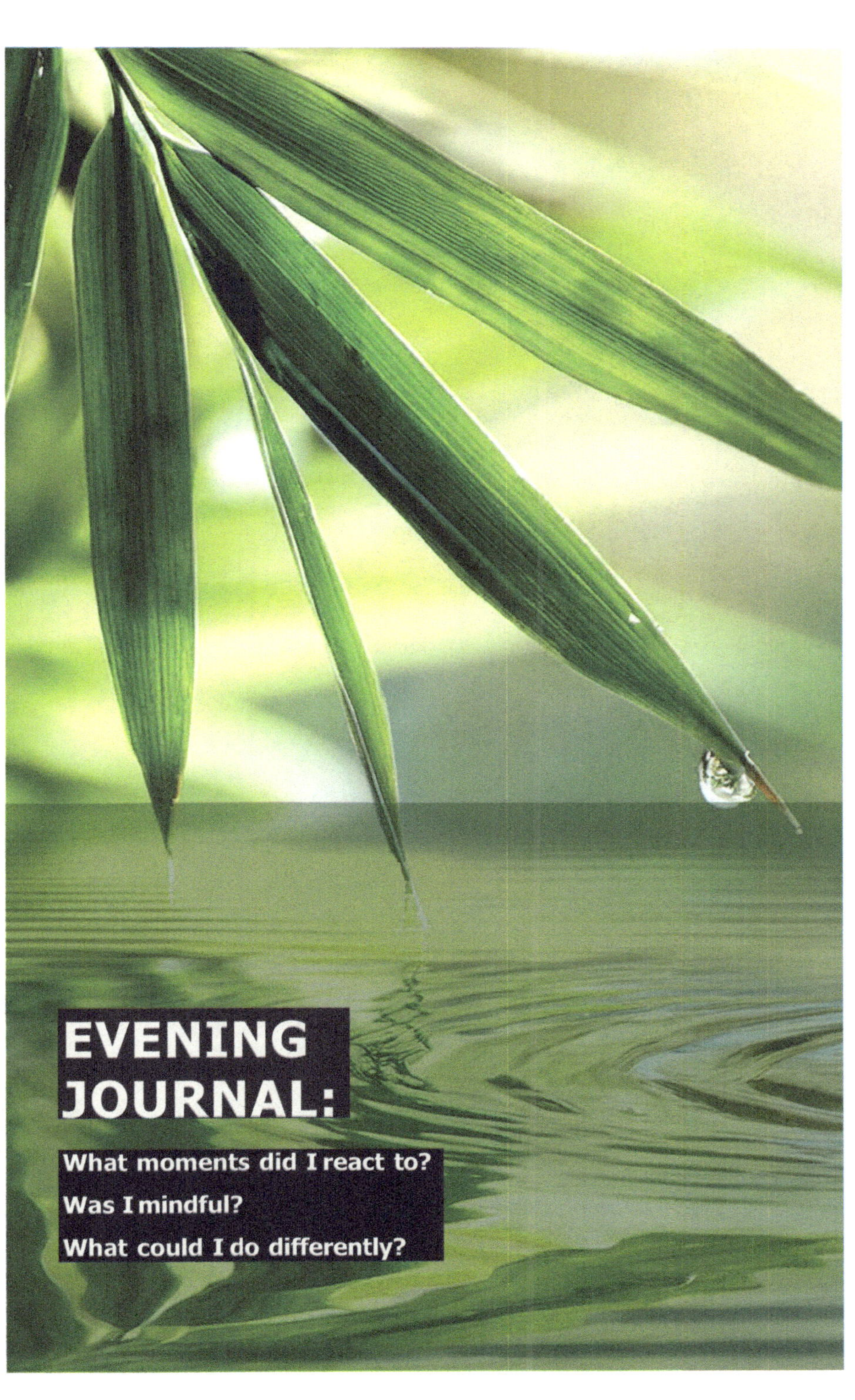
EVENING
JOURNAL:
What moments did I react to?
Was I mindful?
What could I do differently?

DAY 7

FLOOD YOUR BRAIN

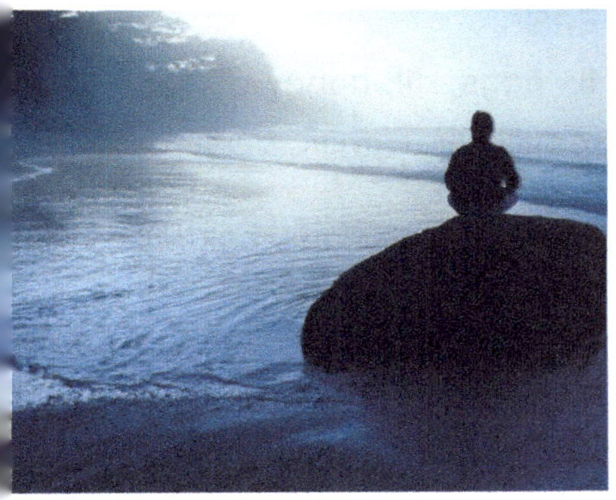

Now that you are finished with the seven-day reset, try to create habits. Don't try to change too many at once. Maybe have a habit theme of the week or month. Create a morning routine to build on your new habit.

ONE FINAL EXERCISE: Go back through your entire week and write down positive influences, great conversations, and celebrated wins. Remember those fun moments with friends. Recall that well-done work assignment. Flood your brain with the good and positive. Help your mind become more aware of the wonderful things about life and overwrite those things that don't deserve your attention.

DAY 7 MENU

BREAKFAST:
Coconut Flour Blueberry Pancakes

Prep time: 10 minutes

Cook time: 10 minutes

Serves: 4-6

INGREDIENTS

- 3 eggs
- 2 tbsp coconut oil, melted and cooled, plus a little for pan
- 2 tbsp honey
- 1/3 cup coconut milk
- 1/2 tsp vanilla extract
- 1/4 cup blueberries
- 1/4 cup coconut flour
- 1/8 tsp baking soda
- Pinch of sea salt

STEPS

- Mix eggs, oil, honey
- Add coconut milk, vanilla, berries
- Lightly mix in flour, baking soda, and salt
- Heat a little coconut oil in pan over medium heat
- Pour batter in for desired size pancakes
- Flip pancake when bubbles appear and cook another few minutes
- Serve pancakes with organic grass-fed butter and either honey or pure maple syrup

DAY 7 MENU

LUNCH:

Rainbow Cabbage Slaw

Prep time: 10 minutes

Serves: 4-6

SLAW

INGREDIENTS

- 1 small purple cabbage, shredded
- 1 small green cabbage, shredded
- 1 cup shredded carrots
- 3/4 cup chopped cilantro
- 1/2 cup sliced green onion
- 1 seeded, diced jalapeño pepper
- 1/2 cup chopped cashews

STEPS

- Shred the purple and green cabbage in a large bowl
- Add the rest of the listed ingredients
- Toss with dressing and serve

DRESSING:

INGREDIENTS

- 4 tbsp olive oil
- 4 tbsp maple syrup
- 4 tbsp apple cider vinegar
- 4 cloves minced garlic
- 1/4 tsp cayenne pepper
- Sea salt/ cracked black pepper

STEPS

- Whisk or blend all ingredients in small bowl

DAY 7 MENU

DINNER:

Vegetable Curry with Cashews and Riced Cauliflower

Prep time: 20 minutes

Cook time: 45 - 60 minutes

Serves: 4

VEGETABLE CURRY

INGREDIENTS

- 3 tbsp coconut oil
- 1 large onion, chopped
- 3 cloves garlic, chopped
- 1/2-inch ginger, peeled and chopped
- 1 tsp turmeric
- 1 tsp cumin
- 3 peeled, chopped sweet potatoes
- 5 chopped carrots
- 1 cup cauliflower florets
- 1/2 cup vegetable broth
- 1 can coconut milk
- 1/2 cup cashews
- Optional: 1/2 cup of bright green vegetable (shelled peas, chiffonade of kale or spinach) (to be added close to end of simmer)

STEPS

- Melt 3 tbsp coconut oil in large pot
- Add onion, garlic, ginger, and spices
- Sauté until onion is cooked
- Add sweet potatoes, carrots, cauliflower, and vegetable broth
- Cover pot and cook over medium heat for 15 minutes
- When vegetables are soft, add one can coconut milk
- Heat through on low
- Serve over Riced Cauliflower and top with cashews

RICED CAULIFLOWER

INGREDIENTS

- 1 head of cauliflower

STEPS

- Cut one head cauliflower into chunks - use florets and stems
- Place in bowl of food processor and pulse 2-3 minutes, until it looks like rice. Take care not to over-process or you will have cauliflower mash
- Heat (no oil) for 2 minutes over medium heat, just until warm
- Stir so it doesn't brown
- Cover and remove from heat

DAY 7 MENU

DESSERT: Honey Roasted Nuts

Prep time: 5 minutes

Cook time: 10-12 minutes

INGREDIENTS

- 1 cup each raw walnuts, pecans, cashews, almonds
- 1/4 cup raw pepitas and/or sunflower seeds (both optional)
- 3-4 tbsp olive oil
- 3-4 tbsp honey
- Dash of sea salt

STEPS

- Spread nuts/seeds in one layer on sheet
- Drizzle with olive oil and honey
- Salt and toss to coat evenly with a spatula. *Really spend some time here to be sure everything is coated*
- Roast at 350° for 10 - 12 minutes *Note: Watch roasting carefully, nuts can burn*
- When done, remove cookie sheet from oven and immediately transfer nuts to a non-heated cookie sheet so that honey sticks to the nuts and doesn't harden on the hot pan.

Featured Brain Boost Ingredient:
WALNUTS

- Rich source of omega-3 fatty acids
- Contains high levels of alpha linoleic acid
- Good source of protein

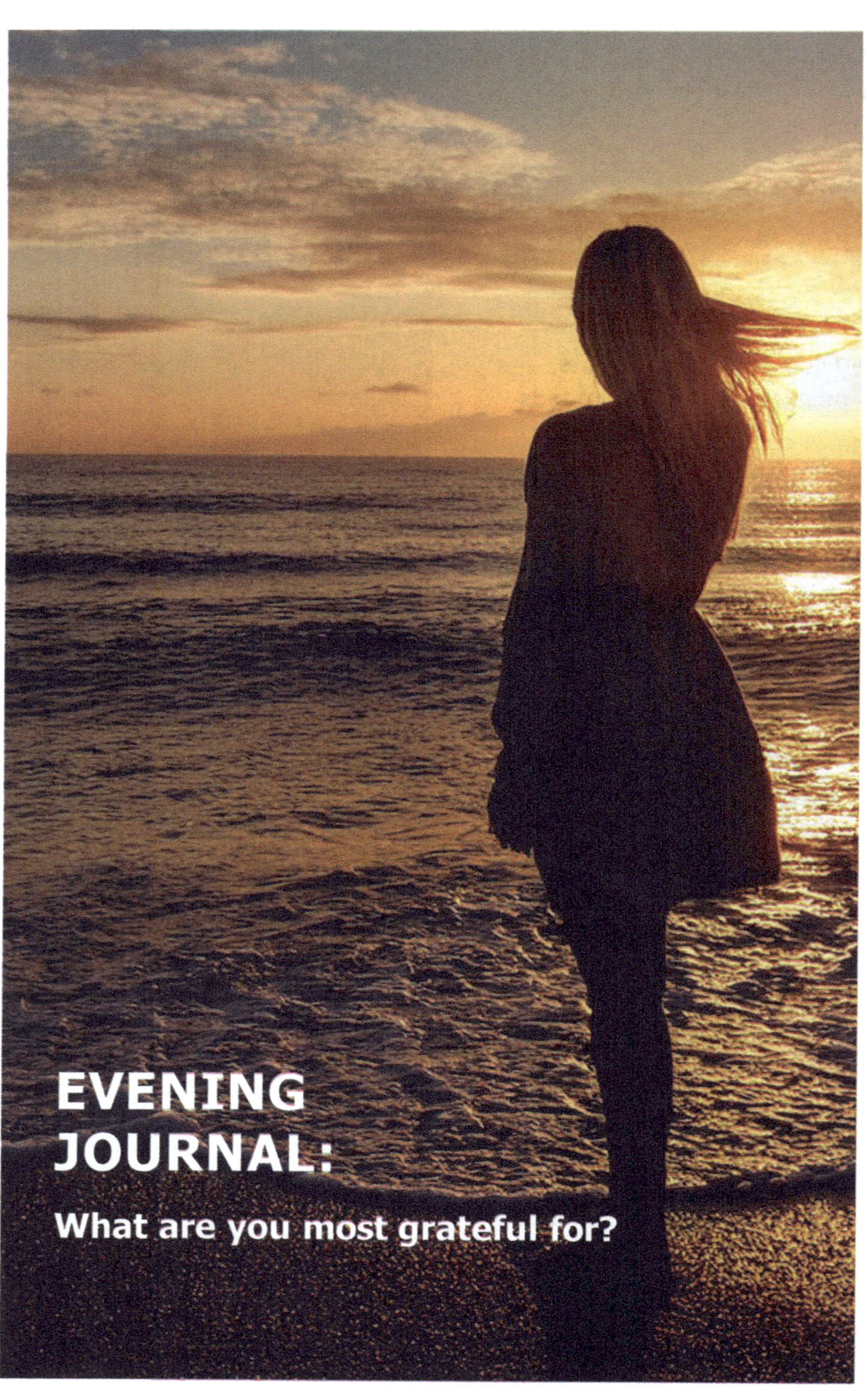
EVENING
JOURNAL:
What are you most grateful for?

THANK YOU!

A book is a labor of love from a big generous village!

So many people helped in so many ways.

One thousand thank yous to:

Jacques Pierre Cole

Francie Rawlings

Michael Molanphy

Todd Murphy

April Bolduc

Delia Garland

Ubaldo Riboni

Isabel Cruz

Sutapa

Priya Ford

Jack Ganguly

And the countless others who shared support.

And thank **YOU** for reading!

Made in the USA
Coppell, TX
18 February 2026

71792622R00069